praise for
things i wish my mother had told me

things i wish
my mother had told me

A GUIDE TO LIVING WITH
IMPECCABLE GRACE & STYLE

LUCIA VAN DER POST

Da Capo
LIFE
LONG

A Member of the Perseus Books Group

Originally published in Great Britain in 2007 by John Murray (Publishers), and Hachette Livre UK company. This edition, which has been revised for North American readers, is published by arrangement with John Murray.

Grateful acknowledgment is made to the estate of Elizabeth David for permission to reprint the recipe for orange soufflé on page 292, from *A Book of Mediterranean Food,* originally published by Penguin Books in 1950.

Designed by Pauline Brown

Library of Congress Cataloging-in-Publication Data

Van der Post, Lucia.
   Things I wish my mother had told me : a guide to living with impeccable grace and style / Lucia van der Post. — 1st Da Capo Press ed.
      p.   cm.
   Includes index.
   HC ISBN 978-0-7382-1278-4 (alk. paper)
   PB ISBN 978-0-7382-1383-5
   1. Beauty, Personal. 2. Feminine beauty (Aesthetics) 3. Women—Psychology.
4. Conduct of life. I. Title.
   HQ1219.V36 2008
   646.7'042--dc22

                                                                    2008030618

First Da Capo Press edition 2008
First Da Capo Press paperback edition 2010

Published by Da Capo Press
A Member of the Perseus Books Group
www.dacapopress.com

Da Capo Press books are available at special discounts for bulk purchases in the United States by corporations, institutions, and other organizations. For more information, please contact the Special Markets Department at the Perseus Books Group, 2300 Chestnut Street, Suite 200, Philadelphia, PA 19103, or call (800) 810-4145, ext. 5000, or e-mail special.markets@perseusbooks.com.

10 9 8 7 6 5 4 3

For my family, who matter more and more as the years go by, and in memory of my own mother, whose grace and dignity in the face of life's adversities taught me much.

Contents

A Note to Readers, xiii

FIVE
〰 home, sweet home 〰

SIX
🌹 *food, glorious food* 🌹

SEVEN
🌹 *perfect presents* 🌹

EIGHT
✿ *fun and games* ✿

AND FINALLY...

A Note to Readers

Let me introduce myself. To start at the beginning: I'm not young. I've got two grown-up children and five very small, very much loved grandchildren (all boys, since you ask). While I'm not too attached to some of the things that come with being the age I am (problems with the waistline, sagging, wrinkles, finally giving up on the notion that I might one day do a long trek in the Hindu Kush), there are, when I count them, lots of good things that come with having survived more than a decade or two.

Firstly, if you've been lucky enough to have lived my sort of life, which has had an inside-ring seat on a fascinating period of womanhood—the arrival of the very first tights, the miniskirt, the power suit, the rise of women up the corporate ladder, at the stock exchange, in the law courts, and up into space, right through to the present day—then you have, inevitably, picked up a few savvy hints along the way. Since it seems a shame for all of us to have to learn everything from scratch, to make all the discoveries the hard way, and to reinvent, so to speak, the wheel, this book is an attempt to pass on some of the things I've learned in life.

A little background may be helpful here: I've worked on some of Britain's most important newspapers, starting as the design correspondent in 1963 on the newly launched *Sunday Telegraph,* just as London was coming out of its postwar torpor and the Beatles, fashion designer Mary Quant, crimper Vidal Sassoon, designer Ossie Clark, and later the Rolling Stones began to transform the London scene. From there I moved to the *Sunday Times* at the very moment that women's pages with their traditional take on family, cooking, home and fashion were reinventing themselves as lifestyle sections, aimed at the new modernist men and women. But my biggest break was to be asked to write and edit the newly launched *How to Spend It* pages of the *Financial Times,* in those days still the parish paper of the City, London's financial district. It was the greatest possible good fortune for I arrived just as the paper was beginning to spread its wings, reaching out into new areas, becoming the sophisticated, international, all-embracing newspaper that it is today, and I and my pages rose along with it, reaching ever wider audiences thus giving me the entrée to more and more influential experts.

From all this you will glean that though I was born in South Africa, my life since I was twenty has largely been lived in London. However, my work as a journalist has taken me all over the globe, mostly to the world's more sophisticated cities such as New York, Paris, and Milan. The USA, as none of you needs telling, is a vast and wonderful place, and it would be impossible for me, in this small volume, to uncover all its many secrets, so what I have done here is to write only about the things I really know about and have personally experienced, which means that it is inevitably rather heavily weighted towards New York, with smaller nods in the direction of the West Coast.

Because of my work I have had easy access to many an eminent expert—beauty gurus, emperors and empresses of the fashion world, surgeons specializing in nips and tucks, masters of the art of cobbling, specialists in nutrition and spiritual healing, fine cooks, top-notch designers, and decorating fundis—and I've learned something from them all. I've also got a bit cannier at sifting what seems like good sense from the hot air and downright fluff. I hesitate to call it wisdom, which sounds so self-congratulatory and smug, but all of us who are lucky enough to live so long (*so* much better than the alternative) do, out of self-protection, garner a little more nous and insight with the years.

Of all the things I've learned, it is that grace and generosity of spirit are essential ingredients to the well-lived life. They add a certain elegance to the most mundane encounter, let alone to life's more major dramas. I don't mean elegance of the merely superficial kind—though that, too, is not without its charms. I mean the sort of elegance that, if we looked into it, we would discover is rooted in some kind of moral code. Kindness is elegant—malice and cruelty are not. Warmth and generosity are elegant—coldness and jealousy are not. Touchiness and being quick to take offense isn't elegant, either. (My father always had a motto: "Darling," he used to say, "never, ever be offended. Only small people take offense.") Social snobbery—which is rooted in a belief that material values, such as money and worldly status, are more important than human and moral worth—is not elegant. Nor is the sort of behavior that finds it acceptable to be rude to those who are ill-placed to answer back while simultaneously being charming to those from whom favors may be expected.

But, above and beyond the inner qualities that make a difference, there are lots of practical tips I've picked up as I've coped with the modern woman's lot in life: too little money, too little time, children I love, jobs I've sometimes hated but mostly loved, a busy husband and his career, moving homes, and trying to keep hold of a sense of myself as life hurtles by. I've made plenty of mistakes and there are lots of things I'd do differently if only I could. This book is an attempt to help others avoid making the same mistakes while doing things in ways that make them and those around them happier.

I've also learned that small things can make a lot of difference. Having family and friends we love and care about is all that most of us need to wake up with a smile. If we can then add some graceful flourishes to that sound foundation—if we can look good, feel well, enjoy our leisure, create a home that's filled with peace and some well-chosen decorative touches, good food that doesn't break one's back to serve, flowers, books, and wine—we're almost there.

This book is mostly about these graceful flourishes, and it covers some of the things I wish I'd understood or known about a little earlier on. I hope it helps and I hope you find it fun.

Lucia van der Post

ONE

how

to

wear

clothes

How to Dress

Women have only two ages—
girlhood and womanhood.
—CHRISTIAN DIOR

It was Oscar Wilde who said that only a fool doesn't judge people by appearances. He was right. How we look matters, for all sorts of reasons. In the Western world we have to wear something every day and, whatever it is, you may be sure it tells the world something about you. It signals—more quickly than a lightning strike—whether we are fun, clever, elegant, shy, intellectual, dowdy, sloppy, showy. . . . You name it, dress can convey all these qualities and more. Psychiatrists say that they can judge the psychological health of a person from how they dress—it can speak of optimism and openness, or of despair and utter hopelessness. Those who don't bother can find themselves trapped in a downward cycle of not liking the way they look, and so they take less and less trouble, and therefore they like the way they look less and less. Then they often pretend they don't care, that it's better not to take part in a competition they can't win.

I've met very few people who truly don't mind how they look. In the course of my life as a journalist, I've sometimes written about makeovers, and I've never known a woman not to be amazed and thrilled when the makeover has been successful. I once took a bolshie, aggressive, overweight colleague—who wore terrible clothes, no makeup, and had some kind of apology for a hairdo—to a makeover specialist (Susie Faux of Wardrobe, +44 20 7494 1131; www.wardrobe.co.uk, who helps professional women dress in a way that is sophisticated, appropriate, and yet feminine). Susie's heart (she told me later) sank when she first saw her, but a few hours later the colleague turned up on my doorstep in a figure-flattering, navy-blue, below-the-knee shirt-dress and good shoes, with her hair and makeup professionally done. She was in tears. Weeping, she handed me a vast bunch of flowers, saying, "I didn't think I could ever look pretty." I nearly cried myself. If she could be transformed, so, I assure you, can anybody. It's good for one's self-esteem. It helps one face the world more confidently. It's good for the gaiety of the nation.

And, what's more, it's never too late. Rebecca, in Anne Tyler's *Back When We Were Grownups,* decided at fifty-three that she "had turned into the wrong person" and that her "loose and colorful style of dress" edged "dangerously close to bag lady" and so concluded hopelessly that "it was too late to make any changes." I think she was wrong. There was—and always is—plenty of time to change, no matter what your age. And it's worth it. Completely pragmatically, one observes that those who dress prettily, elegantly or glamorously have a lot more fun than those who don't.

And much of it doesn't depend on the looks that nature gave you. Some of the most famous seducers of powerful men in history were far from classic beauties. They learned instead to behave as if they were. Take the Duchess of Windsor, who was almost forty when she was introduced to the then Prince of Wales. Lady Furness, the prince's mistress at the time, thought her so plain that she felt it quite safe to ask her new friend "to look after the little man" while she went to New York. Big mistake. Mrs. Edward Simpson, as she was at the time, was no fool. She lost weight, became a model size 34-24-34, discovered which mode of dress suited her newly skinny figure, learned to hide her unattractive hands, turned her harsh vowels into a soft southern drawl, polished up her repartee, studied how to present stylish food and how to please her man. It worked. "I'm nothing to look at," she told the American gossip columnist Elsa Maxwell, "so the only thing I can do is dress better than anyone else."

But I also believe that dressing at least moderately well is part of proper manners. Turning up in scruffy clothes to a dinner that somebody has taken trouble with is rude. It takes the shine off the evening. Wearing flip-flops to greet the president, as some members of Northwestern University's national-champion women's lacrosse team famously did, seems to me to show a lack of respect and to speak of an unattractive bullishness. We've all known women who've turned up at work in entirely inappropriate gear: plunging necklines or skirts that are too short. It is distracting and unprofessional. But neither have I ever understood why you can't combine glamour with brains. The fad of some intellectuals for thinking that their IQ depends upon wearing dreary clothes doesn't seem to me to evince much capacity for rational thought.

I also think that the older you get, the less you can afford to look scruffy or unkempt. The young can get away with it, but as time passes it looks less and less attractive, and in the middle-aged and older it can look downright creepy. Older women these days may well be sitting in the federal courts and on the boards of investment banks (think of Pearson's Marjorie Scardino in her Armani suits; think of the lovely Nancy Pelosi, beautifully coiffed and impeccably turned out; or Martha Stewart, all glossy blonde hair and effortless glamour), or presiding over operating theaters, running countries, writing books, and living full and active lives.

They needn't have gray hair any longer, if it doesn't suit them. Skin-care and beauty companies, nutritionists and personal trainers are making sure that these women are honed and toned, pampered and groomed. Glamour is a great life enhancer, and there's no need to surrender it simply because the years are rolling by. Nor does it depend on continually buying loads of new clothes. A great haircut, fabulous shoes, cute bags, and jewelry (which does *not* have to be expensive) all can do much to add more than a touch of glamour.

There's no need to copy fashion blindly, either. I'm of the view that the older you get, the more quietly you should follow fashion—follow it, of course, but at a distance. Wear diluted versions of the hot looks. And I believe in the dictum of Diana Vreeland, the legendary editor of *Harper's Bazaar:* "The greatest vulgarity is any imitation of youth and beauty." Which brings me to honesty—an essential element of real style. What is vulgar and inelegant in imitating youth and beauty (which is entirely different from wanting to look your best) is that it is dishonest, it is trying to pretend that things are other than they are.

I don't think there has ever been a better time for women wanting to look their best. It takes a modicum of time and money, but then, doesn't everything that is worthwhile? I like to remind myself of the words of Luciana Avedon, wife of the famous photographer Richard Avedon, who said:

> *There will always be glamorous women who*
> *declare that they do nothing special to maintain*
> *their trim, attractive bodies; a zest for living is*
> *what keeps you young, they proclaim. I do not*
> *envy them; I just don't believe a word they say.*
>
> —LUCIANA AVEDON

I'm with Luciana Avedon. Glamour requires work, but the tools are there. And they are to be found in places and at prices within reach of almost all. She was only putting into other words what Helena Rubinstein, the great cosmetician, always said: "There are no ugly women, only lazy ones." I believe that, too.

Finding Your Own Style

There is no such thing as an ugly woman—there are only the ones who do not know how to make themselves attractive.

—Christian Dior

I can't believe I'm quoting Paris Hilton, but she is alleged to have said: "Dress cute wherever you go. Life is too short to blend in." She's right. What a waste of all the fun that's out there to be had. But finding how to "dress cute" in a way that suits each of us isn't easy for everybody. To start with, we're all different. Some of us share the same subgroups of problems (short legs, large hips, round stomachs, no boobs, large boobs . . . you get the picture), but each of us is a unique package, and finding out how to make the most of ourselves generally takes a bit of time.

It also takes a bit of ruthless honesty. The first essential is a long, straight look in the mirror, deciding what is good about your body and what isn't. Once you've worked out what needs hiding and what enhancing, you're on your way to finding a wardrobe to suit you. The art of disguise is what it's all about, particularly as one gets older, when crepey necks and flabby arms are not a pretty sight.

But none of us gets it right all the time. We can all look back and blush at the mistakes we've made in our day. But if we care enough, we can learn by trial and error what suits us and what we should steer well clear of. I know, for instance, that whereas I love dead plain, classy, classic clothes, they do absolutely nothing for me other than make me look like a rather dreary librarian (I'm sure there are some very glamorous librarians, but you know what I mean). I need something a bit quirky or eccentric to look interesting. I need to hide my now not-so-great waist and go for things that hint at the waist but don't show up its deficiencies. I've got decent legs for my size, so even though I'm a grandmother (remember?), I can still get away with shortish skirts if I wear dark tights. I go for curvy jackets that make it seem as if my waist goes in and dresses that have either a slightly high (empire or princess line) waist or a low one.

> ☞ *Every wardrobe needs one divine dress (mine is in brilliantly cut black jersey, with long sleeves, a deep V-neck, and a curving, long, quirky skirt, by the Turkish designer Ischiko) that always looks good even on days when you don't feel so good.*

If we're great beauties, we can probably get away with a slightly slapdash approach. I do know (very) few women who are such raving beauties that you never notice the clothes. Most of us aren't so blessed. We have to make the best of what the good Lord has given us. This is where personal style and a touch of élan come in. If you look carefully at women who have great personal style, it goes on serving them well into late middle and old age (think of the late Diana Vreeland, Coco Chanel, Audrey Hepburn, Babe Paley, Jackie Onassis, or Helen Mirren). What we see is that somehow at some stage they evolved a personal way of dressing and of being. They develop, if you like, a trademark that is all their own. Style, as one of my first editors, the late Ernestine Carter, fashion editor of the *Sunday Times,* once wrote, "has nothing to do with youth . . . or age . . . or sex. . . . It has nothing to do with class or color . . . or money. . . . It shows in small ways as well as big. . . . Style is personal. It is what is worn . . . as well as the way it's worn." And most devastatingly of all, she went on to say, "Style is like charm . . . you either have it or you don't." It certainly isn't dependent on beauty or conventional looks.

Diana Vreeland was no beauty but, my goodness, she had style. She piled on the bracelets. Wore the high-necked black sweaters. Patted on the pale, almost Kabuki-like makeup and slashed her lips red. When she entered a room you noticed it. She was a living example of the fact that if you make a style your own, if you believe in it and wear it with confidence, others will believe in it too. Coco Chanel cropped her hair short, came up with a new liberating uniform of soft jersey trousers, skirts and jackets, and made them glamorous. With them, she always wore huge ropes of pearls (she preferred them to be fake; pearls of such size and in such number would be vulgar if real, but the fact that they were fake removed any hint of ostentation) and her trademark jeweled cuffs.

Those who use lack of funds as an excuse might ponder the story of Gloria Guinness, a legendary style icon in her day, who had been poor in her time. When she had very little money she would buy a beautiful piece of jersey, cut a hole in the top, put it over her head and tie an attractive sash around her waist—and everybody would ask her where she'd bought her dress. Now that is serious style.

When I think of my most stylish friends (mostly well past the first flush of youth), I realize that they are not the ones who take refuge in conventionally "tasteful" attire. They shop at Japanese designers, such as Issey Miyake and Comme des Garçons; they love the Belgians, such as Martin Margiela and Ann Demeulemeester. They go for Shirin Guild, whose loose, slightly arty, ethnic take on fashion is perfect for those whose waist is just a distant memory. If they put on weight they fall in love with Eskandar (who has his own shop down in Manhattan's East Village at 33 E. Tenth St., New York 10003; 212-533-4200) or Eileen Fisher (who, together with Eskandar, is sold by Neiman Marcus and Saks Fifth Avenue as well as other good stores, and both have good Web sites—www.eskand ar.com and www.eileenfisher.com), whose easy trousers and roomy shirts and sweaters make them look interesting. They drop in on Salon Z at Saks Fifth Avenue where they know that their interests are always kept in mind. They believe in a touch of eccentricity—but not too much. While they always look fashionable, they're not slaves to fashion. Many of them do wear a lot of black. They tend to have evolved a style that includes minimalist Japanese clothes, trousers, flattering sweaters and jackets (some of them acquired over time) and they mostly stick to a chic template that is essentially fairly constant as well as being all their own. They've learned that it is better to buy one really amazing piece—a jacket, say, from Miyake or Yohji Yamamoto, Chloé, or Marc Jacobs that can clock up many years of service—than a whole mountain of cheaper numbers that die a quick death.

All these women illustrate an interesting point. The kiss of death when one gets older is to dress in bland good taste. The older you get the less classic you can afford to be. A brilliantly tailored, understated suit may look divine on a slim young thing, but once you're over fifty you risk looking plain frumpy. So . . . unless you're a drop-dead beauty, when you can get away with anything, forget the tasteful understated dinky bits of jewelry, the quiet modesty of the pump, the absolutely dead simple dress, and opt for something much more dashing.

For the young, sometimes a really classy pair of premium jeans, a sparkling white T-shirt, a cutely cut jacket, and some great accessories are all they need. Think Jennifer Aniston, Liz Hurley, and Kate Hudson, and you'll get the picture. The key is that white is very flattering, but it must be clean and truly white. Girly shirts and blouses look good with designer jeans too. Footwear matters greatly; in the winter, for going to the supermarket or doing the school run, boots are fabulous. For summer days, loafers, for those who don't mind wearing flats, look classy. The whole look can be jazzed up with high heels. But you need to start by knowing that you look good in jeans. (For more on jeans, see page 75.)

At the end of the day, though, style is hard to define, but one thing is certain: most of us know it when we see it. It takes in clothes—an awareness of how to dress and how to give one's way of dressing a certain distinction—but since style is an expression of who we are, and it tells the world something of our inner selves, it is also no accident that most of those women deemed stylish by their peers are also pretty nifty at creating attractive homes and preparing lovely food.

If you have trouble finding your own style—and, after all, some of you may well be doing infinitely more important things than cruising the fashion floors—or if you feel your look or wardrobe is in need of a fillip, it might be a good idea to book an appointment with a personal shopper in a good store near you (see page 81).

Don't be predictable—be you.
—NATALIE MASSENET OF NET-A-PORTER.COM

Problem Shapes

Big Boobs: Get a proper bra (see page 48). A shallow V-neck creates the illusion of length. Never wear high, round necks, but you can wear high collars.

Small Boobs: Get a proper push-up bra if you're wearing anything with a low neckline. You can wear high necks and, if your boobs are small enough, even go braless.

(continues)

Problem Shapes (*continued*)

Large Hips: Go for A-line skirts, and skirts and dresses that skim rather than fit tightly. Do not be tempted to wear a tent or you may well end up looking like one. Distraction is the name of the game. Provide interest at the neck—a gorgeous blouse with a fantastic collar, or great jewelry. Spandex is a large girl's friend. Jackets that curve in at the waist and out again make the curves look charming instead of bulky.

Flabby Tummy: Avoid ruched or pleated skirts. Never wear anything too tight. A low-slung waist for skirts or dresses, or high-waisted, princess-line dresses flatter and hide the tummy. Keep away from belts tied around the middle. Invest in Spanx—the perfect answer to the flabby tummy and worn, so we're told, by many a celeb new mother in those anxious weeks before the post-baby flab dissolves. As I write, the "sack" or the "big easy" is hotly tipped as the fashion item of the moment—perfect for hiding flabby tummies. Keep it as short as your legs and decency allow, clad your legs in great tights and you're off.

Large Bottom: Choose waisted jackets that flare out and end below the butt. Never wear those boxy jackets that make even skinny beans look square. Keep away from high-waisted pants. Perk up your top half. Curves are nothing to be ashamed of, so wear something fitted, provided it is not remotely tight. Indulge in diversionary tactics. Keep the eye of the beholder looking up-wards. The "sack" (see **Flabby Tummy**) is great for you, too.

Curvy: Don't dress in kaftans and tents, as they'll only make you look larger. Get jackets and skirts

(*continues*)

Problem Shapes (*continued*)

that fit properly but that skim the curves. Take care with grooming. Get a sharp haircut, neither too short nor too long. Add great earrings or a brilliant scarf or necklace. For evenings, a scintillating taffeta coat in a brilliant color (such as emerald green, claret, or scarlet) over sleek, well-fitting black (either a skirt or pants) can look like a million dollars—Suzy Menkes, fashion editor of the *International Herald Tribune,* does this look to perfection. You probably shouldn't wear flat shoes; a heel will give greater length to the leg, which is never bad.

Skinny: You should be so lucky. You can indulge in fashion's more extravagant notions—large sleeves, huge belts, and tweed skirts. You can do the Carla Bruni number and wear a demure coat belted in the middle. You can also look adorably frail in slightly large clothes. Shirin Guild and Eskandar, for instance, are often thought of as the saviors of the larger figures, but actually look good on the very slim because their roomy styles accentuate the delicacy of the skinny frame.

Bad legs: Pants, of course. Dark tights. Careful assessment of the best length for the hem of a skirt or dress. In winter wear boots under dresses and skirts. Choose shoes that have height and lengthen the leg, and never, ever wear an ankle strap.

How to Dress for Work

The first question has to be: what work? The television industry, for instance, seems terminally scruffy, with jeans and T-shirts being the standard uniform. On the other hand, if you were even the lowliest closet girl at Condé Nast, you wouldn't survive long if you didn't know how to put your Macy's or your Zara numbers together with a bit of verve and originality. And you'd better make sure that your hair is shiny, your shoes up to the minute, and your makeup spot-on if you don't want to be ushered out of the door the minute your internship is up.

But on the whole, the real conundrum is why so many women adopt such a bland uniform for work. While I do understand that wearing an itsy-bitsy miniskirt and vertiginous heels when trying to look like a safe pair of hands for a million-dollar fund isn't a good idea, I can never understand why turning up in dreary clothes is meant to add gravitas to the proceedings. I've lost track of the number of highly paid accountants and lawyers who take refuge in terminally boring uniforms of safe shoes, black, gray, or navy suits (and I'm not talking Alexander McQueen here), and unenterprising haircuts. Americans can be some of the worst offenders, though admittedly they are often beautifully groomed, which makes up for a lot. Look at the women in high political life. Apart from Condoleezza Rice, who looks splendidly and appropriately chic, they mostly wear middle-of-the-road pantsuits with bland jackets (the better to hide the hips and stomachs), sensible shoes and a string of pearls. Where's the fun and the personality in that? It's perfectly possible these days to dress much more zippily and yet still look like the safe custodian of a tough criminal case or a zillion-dollar trust fund. Ségolène Royal, the former French presidential candidate, showed that it can be done. The polls told us that her penchant for a lot of sharply cut, very feminine white suits was a large part of her appeal and though she didn't win the election she won plenty of plaudits for her clothes. Paule Ka is said to be one of the niche brands she often wears.

Great shoes dress up the look of a suit no end, and while I concede they're not great for subways or buses, what's wrong with keeping a couple of pairs in the office drawer or carrying them around in the oversized bags that are the current fashionable tote? Then there's the suit itself. Suits don't have to be boring. Key is the jacket, which should be sexily cut so that it doesn't look bland and boxy. A proper working wardrobe should have lots of different jackets, sharply cut, curvy, with flattering collars and necklines (and, most particularly, not those masculine lapels that you get on men's suits), to perk up even classic black slacks or any number of skirts.

For certain roles (such as investment banking or corporate law) you need to look as if you're one tough cookie when it comes to the negotiating table but a real woman underneath, very efficient yet worldly and sophisticated. Or, as Melanie Griffith put it so memorably in *Working Girl,* with "a head for business and a bod for sin." For which no better garment was ever devised than the pantsuit. But a great pantsuit, not the safe, boring one so beloved of Middle America. Remember how Gucci, under the now departed Tom Ford, did the office-babe look to perfection? All efficient pinstripes, but sexed up with great shoes and sometimes a very girly camisole with a tiny bit of lace showing at the neckline. The trick is to find one that is beautifully cut, that has some curves so that you look womanly and, for the sake of your own self-esteem, also has an air of authority. The masters of the art are, of course, Yves Saint Laurent, who first took the masculine suit and made it seductively feminine, Jil Sander and M. Armani, though Stella McCartney and Alexander McQueen also know how to cut a nifty suit.

In fact a pantsuit by M. Armani should be in the wardrobe of all who can afford it—it can take you anywhere from the toughest business meeting to the most seductive dinner (you just add some stilettos, possibly a lacy camisole under the jacket and a jewel or two). None of it comes cheap, so you have to think in terms of investment dressing.

If you're just starting out on the corporate ladder and don't yet have the salary to fund these labels, you could do a lot worse than scour the rails of Zara, H & M, or Banana Republic, or look out for some of the designer lines at Target. I particularly like Jovovich-Hawk's designs, and you'd better catch Isaac Mizrahi's numbers while they're still about (he's decamping to Liz Claiborne any minute). Search for a jacket that has personality and isn't dull, and team it with the best-fitting trousers you can find.

Dana Buchman (65 East Fifty-seventh Street, New York 10022; 212-319-3258) understands what the city slicker needs to wear to work and does the career woman's suits to perfection at moderate prices.

But the days when the pantsuit was the only real option are over. Skirts have been big recently, and there are lots that manage that tricky maneuver of looking both feminine and pretty and yet suitable for work. Teamed with a sexy jacket and underneath a cashmere sweater, a good shirt or blouse (Chloé, Chloé, Chloé, if you can afford it), they make more beguiling work wear than boring pantsuits. A selection of really cute, well-cut jackets (*not* boxy) can go an awfully long way toward giving you a versatile wardrobe.

These days dresses can go happily to work, too. The days when they only came with spaghetti straps and minuscule sleeves are long gone. I think so many of us complained so loudly that the designers actually listened for once and now we are all spoiled for choice—there are any number of delicious, wearable, and—more to the point—utterly suitable numbers about.

Good Labels to Look For

AT THE EXPENSIVE END
Alexander McQueen does fabulous suits and jackets—very sexy but appropriate, too, for the workplace.

Chloé—blouses and dresses to take out a mortgage for.

Paul Smith—for suits and dresses.

Stella McCartney specializes in brilliant tailoring—she does it to special order as well—and she seems to be coming into her rather fabulous prime.

Donna Karan goes in for understated sophistication and nearly always has great suits, coats, and jackets for the upmarket working wardrobe.

Calvin Klein has been reinvigorated under the design direction of Francisco Costa, and his clean, crisp lines are perfect for the working wardrobe. He has some especially sophisticated dresses—he takes sober gray and makes it chic and sexy at the same time.

Ralph Lauren—but of course—the master at adding a bit of interest to what could otherwise be merely yet another classic suit.

MIDDLE MARKET
Theory has its finger on the young pulse and often comes up with the spot-on dress or the perfect jacket.

Nanette Lepore is a label to watch—often does soft tailoring that is both feminine and yet can slot into an office wardrobe.

Diane von Furstenberg's dresses may be a bit ubiquitous, but she's awfully clever at reinventing the dress and these days does far more than just her famous wrap version.

(continues)

Good Labels to Look For (*continued*)

Anna Sui does great dresses, some brilliantly demure in a kind of sexy-nanny way.

Phillip Lim recently opened his own store at 115 Mercer Street, New York, but is also widely available in other stores around the United States and is sold on net-a-porter.com. His feminine, rather decorous, take on the mood of the day makes him infinitely wearable and his prices, as I write, make him relatively affordable.

MaxMara usually has great coats, jackets, and dresses.

Sara Berman does brilliantly wearable versions of the hot fashion trends and she's available at a handful of stores in New York as well as on the West Coast.

Elie Tahari, stocked by Neiman Marcus and many other stores, is youthful, and if you shop carefully, you'll find well-priced jackets, pants, and skirts that have just the right touch of sobriety added to the mix.

Anne Klein does the working woman's wardrobe as well as anybody at middle-market prices.

Tory Burch has a bunch of stores with a youthful but clean collection of midpriced jackets, dresses, and skirts.

CHEAP END

Zara—for dresses, jackets, and coats.

Banana Republic—many a working woman's savior, and it's often a good source of the small essentials that can make several outfits work harder—the perfect camisole, the spot-on cashmere, the just-right blouse.

Target—keep an eye open for their regular design collections.

(*continues*)

> **Good Labels to Look For** (*continued*)
> **H & M**—keep your eyes peeled and taste buds on
> full alert and there are great buys to be had. Look
> out for the occasional cult-designer collections.
> Particularly good just now for jackets.

How to Be Glam

*Glamour is what makes a man ask for your phone number
and a woman for the address of your dressmaker.*
—LILLY DACHE, A FRENCH-BORN DESIGNER
WHO WORKED IN THE UNITED STATES

Never underestimate the power of glamour. It's life enhancing,
and even the plainest woman can be glamorous. Glamour is
quite different from beauty. It depends a lot on a sense of personal style and some inner confidence, which isn't always easy
to come by but can be cultivated. A great help, though, is a terrific haircut. Do not be tempted to go to cheap colorists or
Tracy in the mall (unless she's extraordinarily talented and just
about to be poached by John Barrett or Frederic Fekkai). A tiny,
but I mean tiny (most of us don't want to go too far down the
Anna Piaggi route), bit of eccentricity—or perhaps a better
word is *individuality*—helps. As does well-chosen jewelry, but
not too much of it, just some stunning earrings, for example,
or a fantastic necklace that works with the clothes you're wearing. For instance, I bought some amazing scarlet amber gob-
stoppers in Oman, which look wonderful with plain black,
fizzing it up no end, but I wouldn't dream of wearing them
with much else (except possibly with plain white linen in the
summer). They'd be too much. But some of this sort of jewelry

can be bought very inexpensively in the mall—just remember, don't be timid.

Sexy shoes (I keep coming back to them because dowdy shoes kill anything stone dead; for more, see page 58) and a good handbag (see page 64) help, too.

A fine perfume—but never too much (it's vulgar and bad manners to douse yourself in a smell so strong that nobody else can escape it). If you can't afford an expensive scent it's worth looking at natural essential oils, sold in lots of spas and slightly hippie shops and galleries, which don't have that horrid chemical smell of the cheaper scents. (For more on scent, see page 148.)

How to Wear Black
(. . . because no matter what's on the catwalk today, one day you surely will)

"Why is it that whenever a woman wants to feel alluring, she reaches for a little black dress? What makes a simple sheath—devoid of ornamentation, the color of mourning—so luminous? Why is it that a little black dress seems so familiar while at the same time so mysterious and seductive?" So asks Amy Holman Edelman in her book *The Little Black Dress,* thus blithely ignoring the fact that a black dress can just as easily make a woman look like a menacing crow, a drab Mediterranean widow in mourning or an aging anorexic. Not good looks, any of them. But remember Audrey Hepburn in *Breakfast at Tiffany's,* I hear you cry, and what about Jackie Onassis, the very picture of poignant, elegant grief at JFK's funeral? True, true, but study the photographs. It's the props that make them. The little black dress is but a chic, anonymous vehicle for drama elsewhere. With Audrey it was the hat, the shades, the long gloves, the earrings, the umbrella, the shoes. Could you honestly describe the dress? With Jackie O., it was the vulnerable, little-girl, pared-down look, the pale visage, and the impeccable hair and makeup that formed the unforgettable image.

Mlle Chanel herself, she who is credited with coming up with the very first little black dress, warned us: "Scheherazade is easy. A little black dress is difficult." As well she might, given that that first LBD was a simple number that would look divine on anybody blessed with a stick-thin figure, no evident stomach and invisible hips, but rather less beguiling on the rest of us.

So what do we learn from that? That if we're going to wear black—and we surely will, because black is the new black more often than it isn't, and it certainly won't ever be going anywhere for long—we've got to learn how to wear it. It needs drama. It needs to be cut either limpidly in soft seductive chiffon or silky drapes, or skillfully shaped to follow the curves of breast and waist, or sharp and chic the way M. Dior did it in his last few brilliant years and Alexander McQueen does it now. Just because it's black it doesn't mean it's going to make you feel like a million dollars, though it will make you feel thinner, a quality not to be underestimated. So given that some day soon you'll be wearing black, here's how to do it so that the total look is rather more Catherine Deneuve than Edith Piaf.

1. **Very sexy shoes.** Preferably red but, speaking personally, I often wear some brilliant emerald-green Marc Jacobs open-toed platform shoes. At night you can do glitter.

2. **Adroitly chosen jewelry.** You could do the Coco Chanel pearls number. Mlle Chanel, you will not need reminding, was scarcely ever seen without them and, when she wore black, she piled on the strings (fake—remember?). Have a socking great pendant right in the middle of the neckline or

pin on a funky brooch. You should probably wear earrings—
preferably to add light and "lift" the complexion. Just don't
do all of it together.

3. **Great hair.** Clean, shiny, groomed, beautifully cut and
tended to.

4. **A cute handbag.** Jewel-like or glittery for evening.

5. **Add another color** in the shape of a shirt or blouse or scarf.
Jewel colors like emeralds, teals, and purples work well with
black. Also, surprisingly, does navy.

6. **Some bare skin** near the face is essential. The combination
of black with high necklines and long sleeves (especially
both at once) looks a little too prim.

7. **Adapt your makeup.** Black drains away light from all but
the most luminous complexions. See below for how to
make up when wearing black.

Makeup for Wearing Black

Black, we all know, is brilliantly chic and a wonderful default
color for when we're feeling low *but* it can drain the color from
one's face. That is when makeup needs to be applied with
greater care. Here is advice from Valentine Alexander, my
makeup guru, on how to make up when wearing black. To
book a session with her, call her in Paris at +33 6 99 63 34 10,
or in London, where she sees clients in a Knightsbridge studio,
at +44 207 956 846 909.

1. Before a special evening, start off with a mini facial at
home. The main purpose is to exfoliate, and almost all
beauty lines, even inexpensive ones, including Boots (some
of whose products are available at Target), Bourjois, Max
Factor, and Revlon, now sell exfoliators, which remove dead
cells and bring radiance back to the skin. If you can afford
it, use a high-quality mask—such as Givenchy's Black for

Light Mask or Guerlain's Issima Purifying Invigorating Mask—but any good mask will make a difference and lines such as Bourjois (which uses much the same research and resources as Chanel), Nivea, and L'Oreal all have great ones.

2. Apply a brightening moisturizer. When shopping, look for those two words on products at Sephora or even in your local supermarket or pharmacy. If you can afford it, the top of the range is Chanel's Éclat Originel cream. Otherwise, Smashbox has a well-priced Photofinish Color Correcting Foundation Primer (it also has a great Web site—www .smashbox.com—so check it out).

3. Use a light-reflective concealer around eyes, on lines from nose to mouth and around the lips, and on any age spots or imperfections. I prefer Chanel's version, but again, concealers are made for every budget. Smashbox's Camera Ready Concealer is a good less expensive one. If you have purplish-blue circles around your eyes (a hazard, it seems, after facelifts or laser treatment), Clinique's Even Better Skin Tone Collector or Smashbox's Photo Op Under Eye Brightener are both good.

4. Apply a well-blended layer of your favorite foundation, an exact match with your neck and décolletage. Valentine likes Bare Escentuals Bare Minerals Foundation with an SPF of 15, but always make sure it is a good match with your skin. If you have trouble finding a color that suits always remember that Prescriptives will make custom foundations to suit almost any complexion.

5. Fix your foundation with a diaphanous light layer of light-reflective powder—Bare Escentuals Mineral Veil is great.

6. Sculpt cheekbones with light-reflective bronzer, like Becca's Frangipani or Armani Sheer Bronzer.

7. Lipstick—for classic blondes, Chanel's Rouge Noir. For mousey browns choose from the Clarins's Jolie Rouge Long-Wearing moisturizing lipstick line—they have gorgeous textures and great colors.

8. Lend drama to the eyes—make them smoky, using Clinique's Kohl Shaper for Eyes in Black Amethyst and a good mascara. Maybelline, L'Oreal and Benefit all do less expensive good Kohl pencils.

9. Mascara—Yves Saint Laurent Mascara Volume Infini Curl doesn't clump or flake but the best inexpensive mascaras are Max Factor's Masterpiece Max or those by Maybelline, L'Oreal, or Bourjois. As to color—for blue and green eyes Yves Saint Laurent's aubergine is fantastic. For brown eyes go for black.

I told you it wasn't easy, but it is worth it.

OCCASION DRESSING

Remember the old adage: "Beware of any enterprise that requires new clothing." I don't believe in buying special outfits just because there's a grand stiffy on the mantelpiece. I've made more mistakes buying in a hurry because I'm going to the races, to a wedding, to the opera, or whatever than at any other time. I often think it's much, much better to spend the money on a terrific haircut and great shoes.

Of course weddings often do need special outfits—if you're the bride, you obviously do, but also the mother, sister, or mother-in-law of the bride may all feel it's an occasion to buy something new and special. For those who can afford it, it's hard to beat the bespoke route, something made specifically to flatter you. I can't do better than recommend Anna Valentine, one half of the duo who, as Robinson Valentine, produced Camilla Parker Bowles's spot-on wedding outfits. These days Anna Valentine goes it alone, and she isn't cheap, because her things are made to measure and she uses fine fabrics, but she knows absolutely how to produce beautiful clothes that are elegant and graceful too. She's to be found at 15 Cross Keys Close, London W1U 2DN; +44 20 7935 2050. In New York I would recommend Jussara Lee (11 Little West Twelfth Street, New York 10014; 212-242-4128) or Couture by Jennifer Dule (89 Fifth Avenue, Fourth floor, New York 10003; 212-727-8700) who is credited with being able effortlessly to bring off designer-like numbers that fit to a T.

A close friend, who married for the second time in her late fifties, got Vivienne Westwood (44 Conduit St., London W15 2YT; +44 20 7439 1109) to make her a made-to-measure dress, and it was a dream. In a gorgeous grayish green taffeta, it had her trademark asymmetrical figure-flattering cut and revealed just the right amount of décolletage: more and it would have been vulgar; a little less and it would have been prim. Again, not cheap, but worth it for the really special occasion. I'm personally also a great fan of Morgane Le Fay (746 Madison Avenue, New York 10065; in SoHo at 67 Wooster Street, New York 10012; and Saks Fifth Avenue) not just for her edgy, arty, but intensely feminine clothes but also for her dreamlike wedding dresses. As for Vera Wang—well, we all know she's one of the masters of the art.

Browns (23–27 South Molton Street, London W1K 5RD; +44 20 7514 0000), offers a special service for the growing number of brides who aren't teenaged virgins. It takes suitable models (mostly dresses but also some suits and coats) from designers' standard catwalk ranges and then has them made up into slightly more suitable bridal colors.

For sisters, mothers, and other female relations of the bride, I think it's hard to beat coat dresses. Burberry's Prorsum line has had some knockouts in the last few collections, particularly its recent gold double-breasted coat with a collar, which could take you to anything from a grand evening charity ball (where I happened to see one) to a wedding, a dinner, or the theater.

Most designers have some really pretty coat dresses in their summer collections. Even our old friend Zara has had a gold-evening-dress-cum-coat, while H & M in recent memory was selling a gold brocade coat for just about $60. I don't know how they do it.

Coats over dresses are another practical solution to the problem of needing some cover-up for outdoors and something a bit more partyish for when everything moves indoors. As styles vary from season to season, one can't be sure of what is on sale at any given time but if you see a great coat-dress combo, my advice is snatch it up.

Horse races are part of the set-piece delights of the social calendar, and cutting-edge design (such as Yohji Yamamoto, Commes des Garçons, or Martin Margiela) aren't what they're about. They *are* about looking pretty and feminine (unless you're prepared to go to outrageous lengths to attract the paparazzi's eyes), and here I would resort to looking at the collections of those who go in for clothes that are pretty, ladylike, and comfortable (Ralph Lauren, Marni in its not-too-hippie mood, and—if you can afford it—some of Chanel). Clearly what seems right in Florida and California will be utterly different from what might be deemed suitable in Virginia or Maine, where charming little suits and matching coats and dresses are what I think would pass muster.

Party Time

This, of course, is part of looking glam. Apart from great makeup and grooming (about which more in the next chapter), here are some aids for adding allure come the evening.

1. A glamorous evening coat is well worth tracking down. You can sometimes find them in ethnic shops. If you find one,

buy it, in velvet for winter or silks and satins for spring, summer, and autumn. Jewel colors look fantastic. I have an antique Korean wedding kimono coat in a deep blue that always comes out when I need to be glamorous but want to be warm.

2. For real class it's hard to beat a gorgeous skirt (caramel, orange, or fire-engine red) in taffeta or silk, teamed with a plain round-necked cashmere sweater and some great jewelry. Penelope Cruz in a scarlet taffeta skirt and a black cashmere sweater made everybody else on the red carpet look tarty. If you're thin enough, you can belt the sweater.

3. A black lace skirt is a great all-purpose standby.

4. If you don't think your arms and décolletage can stand being uncovered, find a lacy top that covers the offending parts without looking prudish or heavy.

5. Other good cover-ups that do the job, without looking too obvious while they do it, are boleros, shrugs, or lace jackets (remember Helen Mirren at the Oscars in her Georges Chakra gown with its lace sleeves?).

6. I like discretion—I think a bit of mystery is much more alluring than too much cleavage or too much leg (as for too much of both, don't even think about it). My "taste" guru, Amanda Platt, has a sensible piece of advice: "You can quite often get away with one slightly trashy thing (vertiginous heels, footless tights, slightly revealing cleavage), but more than one is tacky."

7. If you're in the money, and you're in doubt where to look, the two names who do evening wear brilliantly are Giorgio Armani and Valentino (and yes, even though he's now officially retired, the line goes on). If you're young (for her clothes often mean bare arms), Alberta Ferretti has a fabulous line. If you're on a budget, it's worth knowing that lately Zara and even H & M have started stocking evening wear. I have a friend who found a gorgeous evening dress in a very inexpensive British store, Monsoon, so it's worth trawling the chains before you lash out on designer names.

8. One beautiful silk shirt with a huge, flattering, stand-up collar is fantastic for the older woman. Think Carolina Herrera—she always teams hers with great-fitting trousers or, for grand evening events, with a flowing taffeta skirt. Sharon Stone sometimes brings off the look with a man's white shirt and full-length skirt or high-waisted trousers.

9. A really sexy evening look, if you've got the figure, is a well-cut tuxedo trouser suit—Yves Saint Laurent is the master. To make it work you need to judge very carefully just how many buttons to leave undone on the jacket. It may look better with a lacy or a glittery camisole underneath the jacket. The chain stores are getting faster and faster at copying current looks—remember H & M, which for a brief, wonderful moment sold Karl Lagerfeld's take on the black tuxedo suit—so keep your eyes peeled.

CHEAP CHIC

For years U.K. *Vogue* used to have a regular feature titled "More Dash Than Cash" but I always thought it was a bit of a cop-out because it seemed to assume that only the young were poor—there was never anything for grown-ups who might be having trouble with their cash flow. Now, if you're young and slender, it's really a breeze buying cheap. The best tactic for getting away with inexpensive clothing is to be a size 4—everything looks wonderful. It's once you get heavier, and older, that it's harder to get away with spending less.

It is worth saying that if you are short of cash, it is encouraging to note how few garments some really stylish women have—though those few do admittedly tend to be very good. When I first joined the *Sunday Times* in the late 1960s I was astonished to discover that the dauntingly chic fashion editor, the late Ernestine Carter, only seemed to have about three suits that she rotated carefully. But they were all amazingly chic, they fitted to a T, and were always pristine. Then, I once looked into the wardrobe of Amanda Platt, an alarmingly chic personal wardrobe advisor. It was quite a shock. I have scarcely, ever—outside a third-world country—seen such a tiny wardrobe. There seemed to be almost nothing in it. For the closet voyeur this is what it held: five skirts, some cashmere tops (skinny polo ribs for winter, which it was at the time) and Issey Miyake's HaaT seamless knits, one pair of slacks, a jacket and skirt, an old black Armani suit ("from his heyday") for funerals, an old Donna Karan black dress, and a new Temperley dress, which she wore to every party that Christmas, teamed with a Gucci cardigan. Her shoes consisted of two pairs of Robert Clergerie boots and an old pair of Chanel shoes for dressing up. That's it, folks.

So you don't need a lot of clothes to be chic, but if you're short of cash it's vital to avoid mistakes (because that's money wasted). So no impulse buying unless you absolutely know that you will get lots of wear out of what you've suddenly lost your heart to. Think what your wardrobe needs before you buy and, if you see a garment that you fancy, think hard about how it will fit into the life and the wardrobe you already have. Just remember: simply because something has a high price, that doesn't mean it's expensive, and just because something doesn't cost much, doesn't mean it's a bargain. If it's $20 wasted, it's still money wasted. If it's hundreds spent well on something that's worn often, it's cheap at the price.

I've sounded off already about how great the chains are, but it's worth saying again that you need a good eye and you need to take time and trouble. You can easily buy a couple of tops for $50, which may not be a lot of money but if they're badly chosen and never look good, it's $50 down the drain. Do that several times and you've wasted the kind of sum that would have bought a really classy number.

There has never been a better time to buy inexpensively. I cannot do better than recommend the usual suspects: Zara (a dream, really), Target (in particular look out for its designer ranges—in the past there were spectacular bargains to be had from the lines designed by Proenza Schouler and Behnaz Sarafpour), Macy's, H & M, and Banana Republic. Gap is best known for its more casual wear, for jeans and T-shirts, that sort of thing, but it recently came out with a fantastic collection of soft white dresses, blouses, shirts, and skirts by the fabulous Phillip Lim so keep an eye on what it's up to. It takes a lot of shoe leather to cover them all, but it is astonishing what you can find.

☞ *Learn what you can economize on. Personally, I think chain stores do great plain, classic pants, but it's probably worth spending a little more on a sassier jacket to bring them to life. Try to have one pair of really great shoes and one fabulous handbag, as that'll make everything else look classier. Really cheap shoes and bags are the biggest giveaway of all.*

I'm not sure about secondhand shops. I have friends who've found wonderful things in them but I haven't had a lot of luck myself, outside costume jewelry (which is often fantastic), handbags, and the rare silky blouse. I usually find that the things I really like are not only relatively expensive but they never look quite right once they're home. Obviously, if you come upon a Kelly handbag going for a song, you'd be daft to pass it up, but as a serious strategy for dressing I've never known it to really work. It's only fair to say, though, that for some of my friends their favorite garment of all time turns out to be the one-off brilliant find tracked down in an antique market.

I've had more success with handbags in vintage shops, and those on a trip to the U.K. might like to know that many a best-dressed London girl keeps her eye on Alfie's Market, 13–25 Church Street, London NW8 8DT; +44 20 7723 6066, where vintage handbags are often to be found (in particular there's a fab stand called The Girl Can't Help It, which has wonderful vintage evening bags, costume jewelry, hair combs, etc.) and, as I've mentioned earlier, costume jewelry. Not so well known, though, are cocktail hats—they don't make them now the way they used to.

New York has some fabulous "consignment" stores. These are the stores where uptown girls, spoiled heiresses, and the shopaholic wives of hedge-fund managers and Internet tycoons come to dump their little-worn clothes when newer ones beckon. La Boutique (1045 Madison Avenue, New York 10075; 212-517-8099; www.laboutiqueresale.com) is one of New York's best known but there's also Margoth (218 East Eighty-first Street, New York 10028; 212-988-7688) and Tamara's Pret-a-Reporter (235 East Eighty-first Street, New York 10028; 212-717-2691). I've often found lovely stuff at Resurrection down in Nolita (217 Mott Street, New York 10012; 212-625-1374).

The Elegant Tightwad (631-841-2111 and www.the eleganttightwad.com) is a great organization for out-of-towners who want to take advantage of New York's "consignment" stores. It will take you on what it calls its Vintage Vamp, rummaging among the less expensive vintage stores on Manhattan's Lower East Side.

In Los Angeles you're spoiled for choice when it comes to vintage—Lily et Cie (9044 Burton Way, Beverly Hills 90211, but call 310-724-5757 for an appointment as it's so hot) is credited with kicking off the great L.A. vintage fad but lots of West Coast beauties swear by Decades (8124 Melrose Avenue, Los Angeles 90046; 323-655-1960) while It's a Wrap (3315 West Magnolia Boulevard, Burbank 91505; 818-567-7366) seems to sell the cast-off clothes of the sort of celebs who daren't be seen wearing the same old thing twice. But remember vintage isn't always cheap—the best, the finest have become rarities and are commanding prices to match.

It's also worth drawing your attention to a Web site called Yoox (www.yoox.com), which offers a mix of recently off-season discounted clothing from many of the great designers as well as some new niche names. It also has a fantastic vintage site but the prices there tend to be high, for this is serious, collectable vintage, not mere secondhand clothing.

Outlet stores are a great place to shop. I still own a couple of garments I bought many years ago in New York at Woodbury Common (498 Red Apple Court, Central Valley, NY 10917; www.premiumoutlets.com), the daddy of them all (in particular, a wonderful pair of heavy silk cream summer trousers). There's been much excitement recently as it has got lots more glam names onboard, including the delectable Chloé. Lots of companies organize day trips there—www.express trails.com is just one of many—and they take all the hassle out of the travel.

Some years ago now American-style outlet stores hit the U.K. and Europe. I have a very chic friend who, like her husband, is in the arts field, and so they're very short of cash. She always looks a dream, partly because she has innate taste and partly because she buys much of what she wears at Bicester Outlet Village in the U.K., a very upmarket way of buying last season's still perfectly fashionable clothing at very reduced prices. Check it out: 50 Pringle Drive, Oxon OX26 6WD; +44 1869 323 200; www.bicester-village.co.uk.

If you're in Italy, particularly Milan or Florence, you will be temptingly close to some terrific outlet stores. There are so many that it's impossible to list them here. Suffice it to say that my daughter is still wearing some fantastic Prada shoes, and I am still wearing a lovely Prada evening coat, both bought in the Prada outlet outside Florence for very little some years ago.

The Italian outlets obviously require something of a journey to get to if you don't live in Italy, but you can check them all out on www.italianfactoryoutlets.com and it will direct you to where to find the outlets for Gucci, Prada, Dolce & Gabbana—you name it, the directory will have it.

What Is Worth Spending Money On

These tips come from Averyl Oates, the very fashion-forward buying director of Harvey Nichols—which could be said to be to London roughly what Barneys is to New York—and so she's somebody who absolutely has to know what's what when it comes to looking stylish.

1. A **good coat** is a great investment, as winter is long and it's key to the impression you make. If you can't afford an expensive coat, you can find great trendy coats in the chain stores at very reasonable prices but try to personalize them by changing the buttons, or adding a border to the hem, so that you don't meet other people wearing the same coat.

2. Invest in a **good handbag**—it will go on looking good forever.

3. **Fabulous shoes** can make even a high-street dress look fantastic.

4. **Accessories** should be either very cheap or very expensive. Don't waste money on the middle ground.

5. A **classic little black dress** is worth spending money on as it can be worn in any season and updated with key accessories.

6. **Don't follow trends slavishly** if they don't suit you. Look out for key precollection pieces

(continues)

What Is Worth Spending Money On (*continued*)
that you think you like, and then buy the watered-down versions at good prices.

7. **Vintage shops** are great places to find gems. Many designers scour the vintage shops for inspiration for their collections. If you find the right piece you will be able to wear it forever.

8. A **good blow-dry, manicure, and pedicure** are priceless. They will give you the confidence to carry off any outfit.

9. A **pair of Spanx** is essential under those tight-fitting dresses, giving you a flat stomach without the work.

10. **Try to plan your outfit** the night before, if you are a busy working woman, to save last-minute panic and therefore fashion disasters when you're in a hurry in the morning.

Up, Up, and Away
(or What to Wear to Travel)

First things first: get a tan *before* you go. We all know by now—don't we?—that sun is a big no-no for the skin. As Dr. Howard Sobel, one of New York's best-known "derms" puts it: "If you don't wear sun-protection creams, then almost everything else you do is a waste of time." But to look your best you do need to look a little sun-kissed. Head to one of the spray-tan booths to be found in most corners of the country or go to one of the salons that offer a tanning service. Fantasy Tan has a treatment without strange orange hues or peculiar streaks, but the downside is that you need two treatments in a row for the best results. It lasts for something like seven to ten days—time enough to do a little gentle topping off with some natural sunlight (888-FAN-TANS and at www.fantasytan.com).

Always pack a great notebook. There's nothing to beat the slim ones with that finest of fine paper from Smythson or the Moleskine ones, beloved of Ernest Hemingway and Bruce Chatwin, which have little leather ties and which can now be found in most good stationery stores. Kate's Paperie often has very cute ones.

> ☞ *Always take a fold-up bag for bringing back home the things you won't be able to resist buying. Longchamp makes them in delicious colors and you can get them at every duty-free shop.*

Sunglasses (or Shades)

It's a fine line, when choosing sunglasses, between trying to look fashionable and not seeming to emulate much-snapped celebs. However, sunglasses are essential urban and vacation armor. We need them to protect our retinas from the thinning ozone layer and to shelter behind on the days when we've, er, celebrated a bit too hard and long the night before. They hide the wrinkles and also make us feel better dressed as well as a tad more glamorous.

They should, ideally, have top-notch lenses (according to legendary opticians Cutler & Gross, this means plastic CR39 lenses, which conform to American standard ANSI Z80.3–1986) to protect the retinas from harmful rays and to shield them from glare.

But I think most people seem to take the whole label matter much too seriously. It does appear that Angelina, Kate, Jen, and all the usual suspects have only to don a certain pair and they sell out in seconds—*even if* they're sporting price tags in the hundreds of dollars. At Heidi Klein (www.heidiklein.com), the oh-so-cute store that caters for the holiday needs of the sort of people who care about these things, they tell me that when Kate Moss donned a pair of Oliver People's sunglasses, they were sold out in forty-eight hours flat. The same thing happened when Victoria Beckham was seen shading her peepers with some shades from Dolce & Gabbana. This is an expensive game to play, though, since these sort of people seem to own too many pairs for anybody sensible to keep up with. After the Dolce & Gabbanas, for instance, both Beckhams were spotted wearing Ksubis, a cult Australian brand costing around $380 apiece. And after *those* came the Chanels, the Pradas, the Diors, the Guccis. . . .

Just recently the fad has been for huge—as in ridiculously huge—shades. Subtler types have gone in for vintage. A cult name in these circles is Linda Farrow Vintage, which are sold in the Linda Farrow shop in London's Harrods or in Printemps in Paris. These are *not* secondhand but they come from a cache made during the 1960s, '70s, and very early '80s and which, for some reason, weren't sold at the time. Some were designed for Emilio Pucci, but there are lots of huge, chic Jackie O. styles.

Cutler & Gross is London's most fashionable shop for what is called "eyewear" in the trade, and its branch at 16 Knightsbridge Green, London SW1X 7QL; +44 20 7581 2250, is devoted to nothing but mint-condition vintage. This is where you'll find all the iconic shapes worn by movie stars of yesteryear. Peter Hermann at 118 Thompson Street, New York 10012; 212-966-9050, stocks some Cutler & Gross lines. There are also two great Web sites worth checking out for vintage—www.giantvintage.com and www.klasik.org.

Keeping up with trendy fads is best done through those magazines that specialize in photographing whatever it is that Jennifer, Angelina, Posh, or whoever is wearing—you can then take your pick, but you can be quite sure they'll be expensive, anything from two hundred dollars upwards. At Heidi Klein (see page 35), they simplify the matter each year by choosing just a couple of brands and they have a knack of knowing what's the hot brand of the season.

But you don't have to spend the sort of sums that the latest shades command. Last summer I trotted around town perfectly happily in a pair that cost thirty dollars from a chain and was asked several times where they came from.

A new/old name on the scene for those who like something more subtle is Oliver Goldsmith. A great name in the 1960s and '70s, it has been resurrected by Oliver's granddaughter, Claire, who tracked down the old factory where they are now making sunglasses by hand just the way they used to. These are high-quality glasses, so they're not cheap (from $330 to $370). Find them at Saks.

For sheer classic elegance, no fuss, no show, let me recommend Persols (in the United States buy them over the Web via www.unitedshades.com—if you're in London and want great service go to Isis, 153C Fulham Rd., London SW3 6SN; +44 20 7823 8080). Persols have very good lenses, come in simple shapes, and they're the kind worn by elegant Italian aristos (the sort who don't want to get into the gossip mags). Recently (viz Prince Harry) Oakleys have become fashionable among the young set.

How to Pack

I think there's a packing gene and not many of us have it. Proper packing is an awesome art. This is how Sean Davoren, the head butler at the Lanesborough Hotel (one of London's toniest hotels), who has packed and unpacked more suitcases than you and I could bear to contemplate, does it.

You should start by investing in at least thirty sheets of tissue paper. If that sounds extravagant, his canny butler advice is that you can reuse it many times and, furthermore, you can easily buy it at most good stores. In an ideal world (not mine, but perhaps yours?) you should compile a list of what you intend to wear each day that you're going to be away and lay all the items out on the bed. You should layer the bottom of the suitcase with tissue paper.

Men should start with their trousers and lay the waistband inside the suitcase with the trouser legs hanging over the sides. All shirts, undergarments, and other folded items should be put neatly on top of the trousers. Shirts should have tissue paper in the center, the sleeves should be folded inwards, and a further layer of tissue paper placed over the shirt, which is then folded in half. Sweaters should have tissue paper rolled into the arms, with another layer of tissue paper placed on the outside before folding them in half. After this, the trouser legs (these are still hanging over the sides of the suitcase, remember?) are folded over the top of the shirts, sweaters, etc.

For business trips, men should put flat tissue paper inside their suit jackets and the jacket should be folded in half by flipping over the sleeves from the top of the shoulder to form an X shape. Do all this and you won't have to iron a thing at the other end.

At Anderson & Sheppard, very swanky custom tailors who take some two hundred suits at a time to New York for their annual trunk shows, they use plastic bags to keep their suits looking pristine (John Hitchcock, the managing director, says they buy them specially, but old ones from the dry cleaner's will do). The key is to have a plastic bag that is much longer than the suit. Fold the air-filled empty part of the plastic bag over the bottom edge of the suit, seal this with Scotch tape to keep the air in and *then* fold the suit in half. The air provides a layer of protection around the suit, which keeps it from forming creases.

Women should cover dresses from head to toe in tissue paper, inside and out. These should, if possible, be folded at the shoulders and the line of dresses to keep their shape. Again the key to garments arriving crease-free is to create pockets of air. The toes of shoes should be stuffed with tissue paper (which certainly makes sense if you've spent eight hundred dollars on your Manolos). Shoes should be put in shoe bags to prevent heels marking clothes or ripping delicate silks. Belts should be rolled and placed in the pockets of space around the central pile of clothing.

Women should take care to seal up their cosmetics. Most pharmacies sell empty, small, plastic bottles into which you can decant makeup. Put them all into zipped plastic bags but, if push comes to shove, even an ordinary shopping bag would do. Just make sure there are no holes in it.

One other tip—the editor of U.K. *Vogue* recently went on vacation to Morocco and made a list of what she packed and what she wore. You won't be surprised to hear that she took far more than she ever wore. So—next time you go on vacation do likewise. Make a note of what you actually wear (as opposed to what you packed) and remind yourself when the time comes to pack for your next trip. And in these days of congested airports and hour-long waits for baggage to arrive, not to mention punitive luggage allowances, it's best to do as most frequent travelers learn to do—slim down the wardrobe so that you can fit it all into a single carry-on that you can take into the cabin.

Mehra Dalton who runs Indian specialist travel company Greaves Travel packs for ten-day trips and fits it all into a cabin-friendly bag. She does it by keeping to a monochrome wardrobe of black and white (she has black and white linen trousers and lots of different tops) and adding color and interest in the shape of pashminas, scarves and jewelry. She travels wearing Tod's loafers (which double for sightseeing) and packs one gorgeous pair of bronze Jimmy Choo's for evening and some pretty flip-flops for other occasions.

The Yacht

Since boat etiquette requires that passengers go barefoot, you'll need to make sure your toes are as pretty as they come. Go for a good pedicure. Yes, of course, you can do all that hard skin removing at home (every beauty counter has a line in do-it-yourself products) but there's nothing like a good professional for making nails look groomed and cared for.

You'll also need some other more tangible props. Think about a delicious floaty kaftan for those evenings when you're sipping something white and chilled while the sun sinks like a great big orange. Since "ethnic" is enjoying another of its moments in the sun you can find kaftans and cover-ups at every price level and the beachwear department of almost every department store has them. Some of the prettiest though are designed by Lotty Bunbury, the wife of the doctor on Mustique. She hand paints silk and turns out simple sarongs, kimonos, kaftans, and full-length cover-ups. Check out www.lottyb.com where she helpfully has a Skype button, which makes it easy to talk to her. She also sells in the little shops at the Cotton House Spa and the Pink House on Mustique and all sorts of chic Caribbean outlets. Allegra Hicks, who does them in sophisticated grungy colors, and Ananya are two other very good brands.

Then you'll need a wrap. Buy a featherlight soft pashmina blanket (use it as a scarf, shawl, or blanket). All good department stores sell them though there seems to be a certain brand of chic young girl who makes regular trips to India and then sells them at private parties to her friends back home. If you're in on this circuit it's a great way to buy. The one I use when I'm traveling comes in pretty soft pastel stripes from www.kuljit sidhu.co.uk (which sadly doesn't ship to the United States). Madeleine Trehearne and Harpal Brar (a British woman and her Indian business partner, at mtrehearne@easynet.co.uk and www.trehearneandbrar.com) import the most beautiful pashminas and kashmiri shawls of every kind—some plain, some embroidered. None of them are cheap (they start at $900)— they import only the finest of the fine. They have beautifully photographed, colored illustrations of them and they will also deliver their pashminas to almost any address. Hermès does the most delicious feather-light versions, and Agnona, Ermenegildo Zegna's women's division, does divine lightweight candy-striped and plain versions. Otherwise buy online from www.uniq looks.com, which has a particularly informative Web site.

Gorgeous sunglasses, it goes without saying, are important. In Britain Cutler & Gross do some brilliantly retro ones if you want a change from the big designer names (Gucci, Prada, Chanel, Chloé, et al.) but there are plenty of U.S. sources of cute vintage glasses (check under the sunglasses heading on page 35).

Next, a great hat. This can be hard to pack so you will either have to wear it on the way, buy a fold-up proper panama (which, bizarrely, as I'm sure you know, comes from Ecuador) or look out for one at a local shop when you land. The Australian designer Helen Kaminski, stocked by many American stores, does soft foldable—and, more to the point, very flattering—versions in straw and other highly technical fibers. You'll also need some floaty linen—For those visiting the U.K., Shirin Guild (241 Fulham Road, London SW3 6HY; +44 20 7351 2766, as well as at Liberty) does this beautifully but so does Ralph Lauren (rather more expensively) and quite often Eileen Fisher and, very inexpensively, Gap. Then you need a couple of great accessories. The true luxury hold-all has to be

Bottega Veneta's Cabat bag in plaited leather. It's beautiful, it's perfect—very Jackie O.—and it costs a small fortune ($5,800 in the larger size, $4,700 in the smaller), from 699 Fifth Avenue, New York 10022; 212-371-5511.

Get some great shoes for stepping ashore (Tod's loafers look very laid-back Italian if you're wearing pants), and you're set.

The Plane

Be comfy. Celebrities or the really rich, whose first-class tickets (or, even better, private jets) are secure, like to slob about in Juicy Couture. I like to wear easy pants, either a pair of quite grown-up-looking cargo pants—by which I mean not too much hardware or too many fancy bits on them—or some loose, navy-blue, silky cropped pants I had made up in India teamed with a T-shirt and a cashmere cardigan. Gap's line of "boyfriend pants" (i.e., loose and easy) are very comfortable for traveling, if not very smart, though if you pair them with a good jacket they can look great. If I'm going from somewhere cold to the tropics, I wear tights underneath and remove them before landing. Over everything I wear a three-quarter-length coat, though since parkas have been reinvented in the lightest of fabrics by everybody from Prada to Stella McCartney (who both used beautiful parachute silks), they fit the bill perfectly. Otherwise a trench, if it suits you, would be perfect—or a swinging trench without a belt for anyone who doesn't like tying things around her middle. I never get on a plane without a pashmina—all that air-conditioning. Debbie Moore of Pineapple Dance Studio fame once told me that she always puts her feet in brown-paper bags to stop them swelling up. I've never had the nerve to follow her advice, and anyway I'm lucky in that my feet don't swell up—but if yours do and you can face it, there's the remedy.

If you find airports stressful, check out Holistic Silk (www.holisticsilk.co.uk). Its silk products are filled with "aromatic herbs and ancient wisdom" (the better, I assume, to make all the hassle seem like nothing in the face of eternity). Kit yourself out with their Japanese brocade slippers with magnetic insoles (about $130), which deal with blocked chi; block out frenetic sights with their silk jet-set eye mask; rest your neck on one of their silk neck pillows, and don't forget your silk yoga-mat bag for restoring your karma at the other end.

Lady Bamford (whose industrialist husband Sir Anthony Bamford runs the family company of JCB) created something of a sensation in the U.K. with her elegantly refined collection of clothing when she first launched it some years back. Now her wares are available at Neiman Marcus, Bergdorf Goodman, Richards, and Stanley Korshak, too. She produces the most delectable accessories for those who spend much of their time at 25,000 feet—she offers a chic suede case that can be bought filled with a cashmere shawl, an eye mask, neck mask, cashmere slippers, and a suede toiletry bag.

Some picky people take their own feather-filled cushions, so if you have one of those delicate constitutions and can't sleep on the mundane ones provided by airlines, buy your own little silk traveling one from the sort of raffine stores that go in for such things—such as Barneys or Takashimaya. Personally, I've got enough to carry, what with books, toiletries, and all the rest.

Now that you can check in online, it's really worth doing. It saves all that worry about where you're going to sit and it means you can get to the airport that much later. You can also—if you're organized enough—get your bags sent on ahead through www.firstluggage.com.

With big sunglasses, to hide the jet lag, and a really terrific bag (here it really counts) that is easy to carry, you can emerge looking great.

The Safari

It's got to be khaki, hasn't it? Though you don't want to arrive looking as if you think you're Meryl Streep in *Out of Africa*—too embarrassing. Since I go to Africa a lot, I tend to buy good khaki things whenever I see them, because you can't always find them when you need them. And however appealing crisp white looks against the khaki, resist the temptation, because when you're in the bush hoping not to be seen by anything wild, if you're wearing white you might as well stand up and shout, "Here I am!'

You'll need good shorts, comfy long pants (often long is best because, if you tuck them into your socks, it keeps the insects at bay), a fleece or jacket and a sweater (those early-morning drives can be perishingly cold)—all in khaki or beige. A few pretty tops for evening and some costume jewelry for perking the look up and that's it. Don't forget a sunhat and a backpack to carry things like your bird book, sunscreen, and binoculars. Safari lodges are good at doing laundry—they turn things around the same day—so you won't need to take a lot.

The Beach

Well, of course, it depends which beach. If it's the Caribbean's St. Barth's, you'll need to look to your smart getup—jeweled flat sandals and ballet pumps, chic black capri pants, easy white linen, big shirts over skinny pants, floaty tops in pristine white, huge woven bags, and great big beads for glamming up. Swimming costumes from Eres and La Perla are expensive, but that's because proper corsetry (which they offer) costs more to make. Lotty B (see page 40) does beautiful silky sarongs and floaty kaftans, or you could go for one of Bamford's beautiful white silk embroidered kaftans (from Saks, Neiman's, or

Bergdorf's). Heidi Klein's shop in New York (see page 35) is filled with very hip beachwear all year long, thus neatly filling a great big gap. Get your swimsuits, bikinis, cover-ups, sunglasses, sunhats, and a big beach tote, all under one roof.

If you are in despair over swimwear, Lands' End, that Waspy brand, will sort you out. It uses Slendertex, a light but fine supporting material, and has swimsuits with tummy control panels, high necks or waist-flattering styles, and even—for those who've had breast cancer—special mastectomy suits. Its amazing Web site (www.landsend.com) has a marvelous section called "anxiety zones" where you can click on your particular problem (big boobs, pear shape, or whatever) and up will come a range of suggestions, such as little skirts to cover the tops of thighs of the heavy hipped, or panels to hold in lumps and bumps, and it stocks some styles up to size 26. I've had women readers in tears of gratitude for the tip. Get a catalog by calling 800-963-4816.

The City Weekend

This assumes a city weekend in what's laughingly known as a "temperate climate" (i.e., northern Europe, New York, San Francisco . . .). Unless you're in the private-jet set, this means serious discipline, particularly with airlines getting tougher about luggage by the day. I've partly solved the problem by settling on one pair of pants, which I team with three different jackets to give me three separate looks. I have a brilliant soft feminine navy blue crepe jersey jacket and pants by the dear, late-lamented Jean Muir. It's very chic, but comfortable enough for flying. Under the jacket, I wear a soft, navy silky top, but if it were very cold I could put on a navy cashmere sweater instead. A sassy cropped navy jacket with taffeta cuffs and taffeta lapels (instead of the crepe jersey jacket) turns the outfit into evening wear. I add jewelry, some sexy shoes, and I'm ready for dinner, the opera, whatever. To make it look different the next day, I wear a sharp lime green jacket in an identical cropped, sassy shape over the navy trousers and silky top. Now the Jean Muir label has very sadly disappeared, but you can easily replicate the solution by searching for an attractive pantsuit and then buying separate jackets (everybody, and I mean everybody, on the high street does them now in very cute shapes and colors). The great thing about this plan for a capsule wardrobe is that it needs just two pairs of shoes (one pair does the day look and another turns on a bit of style come the evening).

Over it, of course, goes a coat, which will vary depending upon the time of year. In winter it's heavier; in summer I choose something more like a raincoat or one of the newly fashionable lightweight parkas.

To give even greater variety you could pack a couple of other tops, possibly one of Chloé's delicious floaty smocks, if you can afford it, or otherwise one of Zara's charming numbers, and a skirt. But for shopping, museum viewing, and city touring, comfortable shoes have to be the nonnegotiable accessory. Tod's loafers are great. I personally think wearing sneakers is pretty tacky, but you can get away with tennis shoes (either Converse or the French brand Bensimon, www.bensimon.com, which is terrific).

Snow

Designer skiwear seems to me to come at preposterous prices for those who aren't married to hedge-fund managers (Chanel skis, I ask you—as if the snow can tell), but really cheap options aren't easy to find. Which isn't to say that if you *are* married to a hedge-fund zillionaire, you won't look awfully pretty posing outside your private chalet in Chanel, Ralph Lauren, Armani, Prada, et al. It's just that for the rest of us, there are cheaper options.

If you're really feeling stretched (skiing holidays don't come cheap), you'll just have to be energetic and keep an eye open for sales and look for the cheaper brands, but since skiwear has to be functional—it has to keep out the wet and the snow— you can't afford to compromise. The fancy brands are mostly for those who spend more time promenading around the resort's smartest shops than perfecting their parallels. Many chain stores these days often sell skiwear or, more precisely, parkas that fit the purpose. The North Face and Patagonia are both good middle-range brands and Lands' End always has great cold-weather gear. Eastern Mountain Sports does sturdy skiwear at very good prices. You could choose an all-in-one ski suit (they may look glamorous but they're devilishly impractical) but fashions in recent years have turned back to the more retro look of the pants and parka option. You'll also need proper ski socks, which provide warmth as well as a buffer between your feet and the unyielding surfaces of the ski boot, and proper ski gloves that have linings and real insulation, and are waterproof (no, delicate cashmere won't do). Proper thermal underwear—long johns and a long-sleeved vest—are vital. Get them from www.figleaves.com.

For skiing in really cold places, I have a neck warmer and a warm hat. And when heli-skiing in British Columbia, I found foot and hand warmers (little packs with magic contents that warm up when you open them, to be put inside your boots and gloves) miraculous. Don't forget great but efficient sunglasses (you must protect your eyes against UV rays, which when reflected off the snow can damage the retina) and goggles for those nasty days.

UNDERPINNINGS

Since delectable underwear doesn't seem to be the American woman's birthright—unlike French and Italian women, whose streets and stores are awash with delicious little bits of nothing—you'll have to make an effort to find it. But things are getting better. We should all genuflect in the direction of Victoria's Secret, which has brought a decent array of pretty underwear to every corner of the land. Visitors to the U.K. in search of proper underwear might like to know that Marks & Spencer now has one of the most comprehensive selections around, and you'd have to be a dull bird not to find something to suit. Besides divine bits of frippery with matching sets of bras and pants, its Magic Knickers are fabulous for days when you want to wear a clingy dress and need to hide any incipient rolls of flesh. Underpinnings, as we all learn the hard way, are more essential than we think. The right ones can turn a rather shapeless little number into something surprisingly sexy. The wrong ones, leading to drooping boobs (nothing is more aging, particularly as one gets older and boobs seem to get inconveniently larger) and floppy tummies, can make the most avant-garde of numbers look like a shapeless tent.

The right bra is more important than anything else, unless you have tiny little boobs, which may not be great for your sex life or for propping up certain sorts of décolletage, but are certainly an asset when it comes to wearing fashionable clothes. The major mistake that most of us make in choosing a bra is to buy one that is too large around the back and too small a cup. I always thought I was a 34D until I got myself measured professionally and found I was really a 32E (i.e., smaller in the back, larger in the cup). Real support comes not from the bra straps but from a good fit around the back. Some 60 percent of women, say the surveys, are wearing the wrong-sized bra. Playtex recently launched a new idea: bras that go up in half sizes for all those who are neither exactly one size or the other. Very useful.

☞ *The Web site www.figleaves.com offers lots of great information on bras, how to choose them, how to measure yourself, and how to make sure they fit.*

Lacy underwear makes one feel deliciously feminine, but it doesn't provide a smooth silhouette. Under T-shirts you need the right size of seamless bra in a skin tone (not white). If you really feel you've gone to seed around the middle, then all-in-one bodysuits are great if you want to wear something like a Diane von Furstenberg or an Issa wraparound jersey dress where every little roll shows.

Delicious underwear is good for one's morale, and anything that doesn't come in a pack of three has to be good news. These days there are more delightful underwear shops around than ever before and that great Italian underwear chain Intimissimi—the patron saint of those who love glamorous undies but can't afford Agent Provocateur or Myla prices—has opened in Columbus, Ohio, of all places—but you can also find some of their bras and panties at Victoria's Secret.

I don't think one needs masses of bras unless one has an extraordinary variety of necklines to cope with. For most of us what we need is: one cotton bra in white, one black in Tactel for wearing under the tightest tops, one nude, and one multistrap (for strange-shaped necklines and halters). Then you need a divinely pretty one for those days when . . . you never know what may happen. And two pairs of matching underwear in your preferred shape to match each bra (as Grandma always said—you never know when you're going to be run over).

Under see-through or white shirts, wear a nude bra, not a white one. Nude Hanro camisoles are perfect for wearing under lightweight tops to give a better line. Hanro is a brilliant name to look out for if you need very, very fine underwear of the highest quality.

As for thongs, I can't imagine who thought them up, but if you like wearing them . . . fine. Me? I think they're about the most uncomfortable and hideous items I've come across in a long time.

When it comes to tights, it goes without saying—doesn't it?—that opaque tights are what you wear if your legs aren't great. Gray with a slight sheen makes a great change from black. In summer, when opaque tights no longer cut it, you need to take care over the precise cut-off point of the hem of your skirt. Wild colored tights can work if carefully chosen; I've seen purple ones look amazing with black and even red. One great beauty, no longer young, came to dinner recently wearing a black dress and wild tights in red and cream stripes with red shoes. She looked fantastic. Such eccentricity needs a really good eye if it is to work. But a lot of pattern only works on *very* slim legs, and even then it needs to be carefully teamed with everything else. The Wolford brand (www.wolford.com) may be more expensive than most but in my experience their tights last longer and have a knack of providing just the color and texture the season requires. Fogal is another brand that always delivers on the right colors and high quality.

If you have areas that need to be corralled in, the name to remember is Spanx (even Gwyneth, we are reliably told by those magazines that specialize in such tidbits, has worn them on occasion), which has all sorts of shapes for controlling different parts. You can get just bottoms or underwear with long panels to hold in the thighs, or all-in-ones for the big night when you want the whole torso to look taut and firm. The Spanx Hide & Sleek Hi-Rise Body Smoother, for instance, starts just below the bra line and goes all the way down to midthigh, smoothing down the bulging bits and cinching in the waist. A name to conjure with. You can find them at lots of stores with good underwear departments. Online you can get them from figleaves.com. Agent Provocateur has a sexier alternative, a girdle that is made from duchesse satin and is more like an old-fashioned corset, pulling in the waist.

☞ *A reminder—Bodas (www.bodas.co.uk), a great British source of every-day underwear in fine cotton, warns that we shouldn't use fabric softener when we wash underwear that contains Lycra—it rots it. Worth knowing that.*

Specialist Shops Around the World

A few great underwear stores not to miss:

NEW YORK

Bra Smyth, 905 Madison Avenue, New York 10021; 212-772-9400; www.brasmyth.com, has over fifteen hundred bras in stock and it prides itself on being able to make sure that nobody who is seriously interested in a proper bra leaves dissatisfied. Its assistants will assess, fit, and advise, alter, and custom make.

Kiki de Montparnasse, 79 Greene Street, New York 10012; 212-965-8150, is the latest destination for the downtown set. Described as somewhere between "lingerie store, high-end sex store, and boudoir lounge," it offers luxurious underwear and nightwear and, though distinctly on the naughty side, there's not a hint of seediness.

La Petite Coquette, 51 University Place, New York 10003; 212-473-2478; www.thelittleflirt.com, is a legendary Manhattan lingerie shop (rumor has it that Sarah Jessica Parker is among its fans) and that will put you right on bra sizes (there's

Lingerie Web Sites

www.figleaves.com has almost every great brand you can think of, as well as Playtex's very new bras that go up in half-sizes. It also has an excellent eight-step guide to finding the right size bra for you.

www.mytights.com is a brilliant site for all sorts of fashion brands that otherwise you'd have to track down in specialist shops. Besides control-top, extralong and petite tights and stockings, there are tights for flying (to help with the circulation), footless tights, and those wonder pants—Spanx.

www.myla.com offers tiny confections of delicious silk and satin for those who want something sweet and sexy rather than more serious upholstery.

nothing like a professional to help get it right), find you all manner of "supporting" stars but also sell you some of the flirtiest, most deliciously seductive underwear around. It stocks a large range of niche brands (Hanky Panky, Prima Donna, and Cosabella, to name but three) but also has a good Web site.

Mixona, 262 Mott Street, New York 10012; 646-613-0100, is a large, cool shop devoted to nothing but delectable underwear.

37=1, 37 Crosby Street, New York 10013; 212-266-0067, was drawn to my attention by the lovely Grant Thatcher (editor in chief of *Luxe* guides) and what a treasure it is—filled with diaphanous silks fashioned into the most delicious panties, slips and bras and even beautifully-made '20s-style dresses. Designer Jean Yu also makes to measure and her faithful clientele seem to have no trouble coming up with the $350 they have to part with for a single pair of panties.

Agent Provocateur has lots of shops—check them out on www.agentprovocateur.com. You don't go to them for serious support underwear; you go for delicious silky creations, all lacy, frothy, and fabulous. They also have lots of wittily naughty-sounding things like Maitresse Body Wash and candles called Strip or Tease.

Victoria's Secret, www.victoriassecret.com, is the working girl's playground. There are branches everywhere and, if it isn't having too vulgar a moment (always a risk), a great place for inexpensive, delightful fripperies. It also stocks some of Intimissimi's (the brilliant medium-priced Italian brand—remember?) lines.

LONDON

Carine Gilson, 12 Lowndes Street, London SW1X 9EX; +44 20 7823 1177; www.carinegilson.com. Her specialty is making the most divine underwear to order. She uses silk from Lyons and handmade Chantilly lace from Calais, and she turns out ravishing bras, panties, slips, and negligees. But she also does swimwear, using the same corsetry techniques.

Coco de Mer, 23 Monmouth Street, London WC2H 9DD; www.coco-de-mer.co.uk. Sam Roddick (daughter of the late Anita) has created a rich, sensual, fun place to buy some lovely—and some extraordinary—underwear. She sells vintage-inspired silk knickers, bras, petticoats, and nightwear, but check them all out carefully because sometimes there are some extraordinary erotic surprises lurking among the apparently blameless pieces. There are also erotic accessories and some really delicious lotions and potions.

Rigby & Peller, 2 Hans Road, London SW3 1RX; www.rigbyandpeller.com. Only lissome young things can get away with itsy-bitsy pieces of underwear. Postchildbirth and once the years start to pile up, proper underwear makes all the difference. Rigby & Peller is the place to turn to once things begin to droop. There are fantastic collections that provide support and a touch of allure for the sake of morale. Things aren't cheap, but they will fit you properly—and it's worth getting your bra size checked out professionally every five years or so. They say that some 80 percent of their customers turn up wearing the wrong-size bra.

Intimissimi, 90–92 Oxford Street, London W10 1DY; +44 20 7637 49550; www.intimissimi.com, has just arrived in the U.K., to the great excitement of those who used to have to go to Italy to buy its wares. It's many a young girl's favorite lingerie store of all time.

PARIS

Sabbia Rosa, 71–73 rue des Saints-Pères, Paris 75006; +33 1 45 48 88 37, (one of Sofia Coppola's favorite Paris shops), is like a divine boudoir filled with deliciously soft silky bits of underwear. Underwear for honeymoons.

Rykiel Woman, 4 rue de Grenelle, Paris 75006; +33 1 49 54 66 21. A special project of Nathalie Rykiel, daughter of Sonia, this is a Parisian take on our very own Coco de Mer, i.e. lots of delicious erotic underwear (anyone for pink silk whips?) as well as some wonderfully useful silk jersey workout pants, cashmere wraps, sweet knickers, and the like.

Carine Gilson, 18 rue de Grenelle, Paris 75007; +33 1 43 26 46 71. She does divinely luxurious couture lingerie but there are always some ready-to-wear numbers that you can take away on the spot.

ONE'S CHAPEAU (. . . OR ALL YOU NEED TO KNOW ABOUT HATS)

I'm a great believer in the power of the hat. David Shilling (who now only makes hats for special commissions) used to say, "The whole point of a hat is to make its wearer look beautiful." My sentiments precisely, though I like Miss Piggy's addition of allure and mystery. Miss Piggy, fans will remember, thought: "One's *chapeau* provides the perfect opportunity for a profound fashion statement. Your hat should not merely say, 'Here is my head,' but rather it should convey a sense of allure, mystery, even intrigue. Here *moi's chapeau* [this under a picture of a rather large black sombrero-style felt, tipped at a jaunty angle] is saying, '*Oui,* I have time for one quick chocolate malted in that café with the umbrellas that have tables on their handles, but then I must board the Oriental Express for a rendezvous with the Duke of Candelabra in the lovely, yet sinister, Kingdom of Rutabagia.'" Miss Piggy had the right idea. A hat that can deliver all that is well worth the hundreds that a bespoke hat costs today.

The right hat can be a bit of magic, which we sometimes need to be reminded of. I like the story of the customer who complained to that great master, Christian Dior, that the price for a hat he'd proposed was exorbitant, given that it was merely a bit of tulle and some feathers. The master took the hat apart, gave the customer the materials and said with a grave bow, "The materials, madame, are free, it is the genius that costs."

Cozmo Jenks on How to Choose a Hat

You must try on lots, even ones you think may not suit you. Remember, you can always take it off. Then there are a few rules: never have a brim that is wider than your shoulders and most especially not if you're wearing a short skirt. If you have a short neck, choose an upturned or asymmetrical brim. If you have a nose you'd rather not draw attention to, choose a shallow crown. Experiment with the angle, particularly with berets, where angle is all.

Philip Treacy, generally acknowledged to be Britain's greatest milliner, is a genius and a master craftsman, the modern equivalent of a Dior. He changed the way we looked at hats. "Hats," he said, "were associated with old ladies and I thought that was crazy. Everyone has a head [observant fellow], so everyone has a possibility to wear a hat." People, he also noticed, feel better for wearing a hat, which is true, too. It's hard to get a handle on the cost of a bespoke Philip Treacy hat from his atelier (69 Elizabeth St., London SW1W 9PT; +44 20 7824 8787; www.philiptreacy.co.uk), though anecdotally it seems to vary from about $1,200 to $6,000, let alone be sure of getting the personal attentions of Philip Treacy himself (he travels a great deal). However, you can buy into some of his magic by getting one of his line of occasion hats at department stores such as London's Selfridges and Harrods. It's worth keeping an eye on eBay where there's nearly always a good selection of his hats on sale. Prices start at about $300.

Otherwise, I love the minimalist refinement of **Patricia Underwood**'s hats. They're elegance personified, and they're made in the finest, most divine straw and—in winter—sometimes in felt, in simple but beguiling shapes. You can buy them at her boutique in Bergdorf Goodman on Fifth Avenue. But it's not so well known that she does a diffusion (i.e., cheaper) line called So Patricia, which is sold in all sorts of cheap and cheerful outlets (Sears for one)—so keep your eyes skinned.

Cozmo Jenks (21 New Quebec Street, London W1H 7SA) offers a bit more razzmatazz (perfect for mothers of the bride), which is no doubt why Jay Kay of Jamiroquai, Kylie Minogue, and Leah Wood, among many others, seek her out. She'll make you a hat from scratch to suit your face or outfit for something like $1,200 and upward (call +44 20 7258 0111 for an appointment). She also does ready-to-wear hats (they're all blocked in a

British factory in Luton, but every one is hand trimmed in her studio), ranging in price from $570 to $1,150.

Marie Mercie has a cute hat shop at 8 Knightsbridge Green, London SW1X 7QL; +44 20 7589 7534, where they'll make you a brilliant little cocktail hat to order.

A new hatter to watch is **Katharine Goodison**, who used to be a lawyer and now does wonderfully innovative bespoke hats. Call +44 20 7828 6498 for an appointment.

At the cheaper end, remember that many a designer does diffusion or ready-to-wear ranges, and good department stores— in the U.K., Fenwick of New Bond Street, Peter Jones, Self-ridges, and Harrods; and in the United States, Bloomingdale's and Saks Fifth Avenue—carry these at infinitely more user-friendly prices.

In the United States, good names to look out for are **Eric Javits** who does elegant, simple shapes and can be found in places like Neiman Marcus and Saks Fifth Avenue, and the Australian hat designer **Helen Kaminski**, who is also sold by both Neiman's and Saks, does very simple fine straws that pack flat (so useful for summer vacations).

The very smart East Coast crowd go to **Suzanne Couture Millinery** at 27 East Sixty-first Street, New York 10021; 212-593-3232, for the sort of hats that you need to wow your fellow guests at weddings or the races.

Lisa Shaub Fine Millinery, 232 Mulberry Street, New York 10012; 212-965-9176, does cute little cloches and berets and is beloved of Audrey Tatou. She'll do bespoke or custom dress a store model.

Leah C. Couture Millinery, 124 West Thirtieth Street, New York 10001; 212-947-3505, is another great little address to know about. She does romantic hats trimmed with net and feathers, perfect for mothers of the bride, or indeed even for the bride herself.

Another tiny little hat shop that many a chic dresser seeks out in downtown New York is **The Hat Shop** at 120 Thompson Street, New York 10012; 212-219-1445.

Eugenia Kim, 347 West Thirty-sixth Street, New York 10018; 212-673-9787, has divinely hip hats, much sought after by the celeb crowd, but she'll also make to measure so you can be sure never to meet another like it.

My young friends, some of whom like to wear gorgeous little hats much of the time, tell me that they get great bargains at both **Urban Outfitters** and **Diesel** (particularly the men's department).

☞ *www.nyfashionhats.com is a user-friendly Web site with some great big glamorous hats for around $150. But these days, you need to know, fascinators, those smaller, quirkier little hair ornaments are increasingly popular, and you'll find them here for around $80 apiece.*

SHOES

Ah, shoes. You will have gathered that I'm rather keen on them. But I've only come fully to understand the transforming power of shoes rather late in life. Of course Carrie Bradshaw (of *Sex and the City*) and her pals cottoned on much earlier. I discovered all this by chance when I was overcome with desire—the only name for it—for a pair of grass-green Marc Jacobs shoes. I bought them even though they were a mind-boggling price. But the weird thing, as I keep telling all my friends, is that in spite of the exorbitant sum they cost—the best part of $800, I seem to remember—they've turned out to be one of the best investments I've ever made. They can transform almost anything—and I mean even the grayest, dreariest sack—into something sassy and fun. I wear them with all sorts of things. They never let me down. It doesn't matter if I'm having a fat day—they still fit. While other fashion trends become increasingly unsuitable (mini jumpsuits, anyone?), shoes are ageless.

So I'm now very keen to pass on my newfound enthusiasm for what the right shoes can do for an outfit. Apart from anything else, they can transform the attitude of others toward you. They can instantly say: ah, yes, fun, sassy, outgoing. Or the wrong pair can equally forcibly spell out: dowdy, dreary, can't be bothered, not fun to know. So think about shoes. Instead of splashing out on a new dress or jacket when you think your wardrobe needs a bit of fizz, think about some really glorious shoes. They're not easy to walk in, I know, but you can always pack them into the huge tote bags that, as I mentioned earlier, are what passes for handbags these days and put them on once you've got to wherever you're going.

When it comes to heels, I'm afraid class costs, and it shows. I wish it weren't true, but there it is. And what's more, shoe prices seem to be reaching the ridiculous heights of bags and to have just as much cult status attached to certain brands. To buy more cheaply you need an astute eye. Target has some good lines, and several impecunious fashion addicts regularly scour Macy's, while Aldo and Nine West (not to mention Nine West's slightly more fashion-forward stable mate, Enzo Angiolini) are always well worth checking out. Zara often has great "of the moment" shoes at wonderfully friendly prices. And if you're living somewhere far from great shops www.like.com will deliver shoes of every shape and kind at really good prices—ditto www.shoes.com.

Keep your eye on the magazines to see what is currently fashionable and then look for the nearest equivalent in the cheaper outlets. Often the difference between fun, funky and classy, and cheap and vulgar is a mere fraction of a centimeter or a minuscule color shade. So be alert.

And if you want a really new, up-and-coming insider name, make a point of looking out for Charlotte Dellal. She does the sexiest, most glamorous shoes in the world. Again, they're not for the timid, but for seriously glam evenings they're sensational. In London seek them out at Dover Street Market in Dover Street, London W1, but it can't be long before they're to be found in the world's more sophisticated emporia.

Every wardrobe should have a pair of red shoes. They have a power and a magic of their own. My own fabulous red pair (by L. K. Bennett, as it happens)—open-toed, with a funky high heel and a crossover strap around the ankle—are my winter-evening standbys. Any black dress is transformed by them. I will never be without a pair again.

Robert Clergerie has solved my winter daily-shoe conundrum. His high wedge heels give me height (I'm only five feet two inches), they're so comfortable that I can walk and even run in them, and the high, closed front made of dark elastic material gives them an elegant look. Judi Dench and Maggie Smith are both addicted to his wedges and he brings out a version of them every season. Robert Clergerie has two shops in the United States, in New York (19 East Sixty-second Street, New York 10065; 212-207-8600) and in Los Angeles (108 North Robertson Boulevard, Beverly Hills 90211; 310-276-8907).

If you want some really cutting-edge, avant-garde shoes that aren't mainstream, look out for **Costume Nationale**. Check them out in Barney's of New York or better still visit their own shop in New York's SoHo (108 Wooster Street, New York 10012; 212-431-1530). Their shoes are quite simply fab, and almost nobody else will have them.

Thanks to Kate Moss, who is often photographed wearing its sparkly ballet pumps, **French Sole** (985 Lexington Avenue, New York 10021; 888-639-7247; www.frenchsoleshoes.com), has become a bit of a cult label. Since their pumps are only about $120 apiece (a mere flea bite when compared with the

These are the Shoes That Have Worked for Me

My wonderful Marc Jacobs: grass-green with platform soles, peep toes, and a whopping great "jewel" in the middle. Yves Saint Laurent has compulsively desirable shoes, as does Prada, but if these are really outside your means (though I do think cheap shoes never cut it quite like expensive ones) then there are other ranges a bit further down the price chain. In the U.K., Kurt Geiger does the fashionable shape of the moment at half the price of the fashionable names while L. K. Bennett, best known for her shoes but with a good medium-priced range of clothing as well, is a boon to the working woman. I also love Christian Louboutin's shoes (Saks Fifth Avenue's fantastic new shoe floor has a good selection) which are incredibly sexy without being vulgar—you can always spot them by their bright red soles—and he does the best espadrilles in the world. At about $230 a pair they seem expensive, but you can wear them all summer long and they come with ribbons, beads, and sequins and in almost every color you could think of. For fancy villa parties they're just the thing. In certain circles Louboutin is taking over from Blahnik and Jimmy Choo as the shoe of the moment and like both those labels Louboutins are vertiginously expensive, but a pair a year is perhaps a supportable extravagance.

prices of Christian Louboutin, who is not many blocks away), customers tend to buy them by the fistful.

Serious shoe fetishists will already know that **Saks Fifth Avenue** in New York has one of the most glorious shoe departments in the world with almost an entire floor to itself and every glam name on the planet there for you to try on. If you want something more niche, a little less . . . well, obvious . . . head on down to **Petit Peton** (27 West Eighth Street, New York 10011; 212-677-3730), which is small but as sexy as they come and packed to the gills with glamorous heels. Or glamorous mommies head to **Hollywould** down in New York's Nolita (198 Elizabeth Street, New York 10012; 212-343-8344—check it out on www.ilove hollywould.com).

Diana Broussard, 22 Christopher Street, New York 10014; 646-336-6365 (www.dianabroussard.com), used to work for Dior, Galliano, and Gucci but now she has her own West Village shop selling her own sexy numbers—as well as her line of jewelry.

Taryn Rose (www.tarynrose.com) is a name worth remembering. She is a charming doctor from Beverly Hills who trained as an orthopedic surgeon. In the course of her work she saw so many feet deformed by bad footwear that she decided to do something about it. Her aim was to create a line of shoes that would be fashionable, comfortable, *and* give the foot proper support. Also, being a very young and attractive woman herself, she wanted glamorous shoes but didn't want to end up semi-crippled. Although her shoes may not be quite in Christian Louboutin's or Manolo Blahnik's league when it comes to glamour, they are handmade in the softest leather and do offer a high degree of chic as well as proper support. She says that for everyday wear, heels should be no more than two inches high. High-heeled stilettos should be the footwear equivalent of a chocolate pudding—delicious but only to be indulged in on special occasions. She also says that if a shoe pinches when you first try it on, don't buy it—it shouldn't have to be broken in. She has her own boutiques in Beverly Hills (9536 Brighton Way), New York (681 Madison Avenue), Las Vegas (3500 Las Vegas Boulevard), San José, and Seoul, but Nordstrom carries most of her range and she can be bought online from www.shoes.com.

Boots: every wardrobe should have them. There are, of course, just two types of boot. There are the warm, cozy type for country weekends when practicality and warmth are what really count, even if from time to time they seem to gain a weird kind of fashionable kudos. Take Uggs, which do the job brilliantly and which many a celeb made—briefly—a cult boot. For practical use, though, some people prefer Le Chameau, those French cotton-lined green rain boots (very chic, from the Beretta Gallery, 718 Madison Avenue, New York 10065; 212-319-3235, but look into its Web site www.lechameau .fr for lots of U.S. shops that sell them).

Then there's the fashion boot. They can come in awfully fancy prices—Ralph Lauren, Chloé, or Gucci will set you back more than $1,000. They're also a moveable feast. Each year tastes and fads change. It helps to keep your eyes peeled or grab *Vogue* at the hairdresser if you want to keep up to speed. Knee-high boots are particularly useful if you're wearing a short skirt, as they make it seem much more modest, which means that as you get older you can get away with short skirts for longer. They're also great—obviously—for covering up thick ankles or fat calves. High-heeled ankle boots, when in fashion, are surprisingly sexy.

Penelope Chilvers is a new cult name in London. Her boots are sold in good shoe departments and The Cross, 141 Portland Road, London W11 4LR; +44 20 7727 6760; www.penelopechilvers.com, but she's best known for her "long boots" (worn by Elle Macpherson, Kate Middleton, and many a yummy mummy), classic Spanish riding boots made of cowhide, with a tassel on the zip and a corrugated rubber sole.

HANDBAGS

Whole theses have been written on handbags and their semiotics. Designer bags now regularly cost more than the monthly mortgage repayment. The current price of the famous Birkin by Hermès is something like $7,500, depending on the leather. I know fashion assistants on small salaries who spend phenomenal sums on handbags, feeling improperly dressed unless they have one of the latest numbers swinging on their arms. They can all tell their Roxys and their Novaks from their Lariats and their Mombasas. Bags, it seems, are the new jewels or rather, as *New Yorker* writer Andrea Lee pointed out, they're like "dowries, signs of possession and responsibility and flaunted power." All this is relatively new. The handbag is no longer a useful, attractive accessory. Rather it has become an object of acute desire, a way in which the "having it all" generation of women reward themselves for all those hours at the coal face. Last winter, a journalist describing London Fashion Week wrote, "Everybody—everybody—is talking about handbags with the intensity of cardinals appointing a new Pope."

It seems to have been Silvia Venturini (she of the Fendi dynasty) who changed the handbag landscape in the late 1990s when she brought out the Fendi Baguette, which turned out to embody in its odd oblong shape (like the baguette that Frenchmen tuck under their arms) the desires of the brand-new twenty-first-century women. It changed the market irrevocably. Prada, Gucci, Louis Vuitton, Christian Dior, Chloé, Marc

Jacobs—you name them—followed in Fendi's footsteps and they seem to have tapped into an ever-widening circle of desire. Bag wars arrived. Some of us, though, are more susceptible to their charms than others. I love some of the designs, but the notion of spending the vast sums of money required to keep up with the latest "it" bag seems to me so obscene that I opt right out and look for little niche numbers that seem to me more interesting, better priced and, best of all, nobody, but nobody can tell where they came from.

I seem to own somewhere between twenty-five and thirty bags, a shamingly large number in my view, but a mere pipsqueak of a collection compared to the true fashionista's pile. Not so long ago the owner of a cult handbag brand did some serious research and found that only two or three of the more than one hundred women he interrogated about their handbag habits owned fewer than twenty-five bags. Of the voguettes, you will not be surprised to learn, none owned fewer than twenty-five, most owned more than forty-five and a few owned more than a hundred. But even in less-rarefied fashion arenas, he found that many a secretary owned fifty or sixty bags, and one middle-aged, very proper PA to a chief executive admitted to having well over a hundred. A secretary, he discovered, would easily spend between $600 and $800 and, if she got a real itch to own something, she'd spend even more. Each season, it seems, women would start thinking quite early which would be the "must-have" bag of the moment. Some kept their bags in the proper "care bags" in which they're sold and, because they had so many and they couldn't remember which was where, they took Polaroid pictures of each bag and pinned them on the front so they could quickly lay hands on the one they wanted (good, practical advice there, I'd say).

🖝 *A new idea is to rent instead of buy handbags. This means you can have a new handbag each month. Tap into www.bagborroworsteal.com, where membership is just $5 a month, which enables you to hire a very trendy handbag at a price that varies depending upon the popularity of the bag, but seems to work out at something like about $180 a month. It is still expensive, but nothing like as expensive as buying them all.*

Personally I like my bags slightly funky. To be sure, I am devoted to my wonderful python Chloé Betty, which rattles with zips and chains—it's great for bringing out when one's entering into competitive fashionista turf. But one of my all-time favorites comes from the shop at the Musée des Arts Décoratifs in Paris. It's made entirely out of recycled plastic and is embellished with strips of Hermès silks. It's made by Luisa Cevese as part of her Riedizioni collection and it cost something like $350. But I can't take it everywhere. In designery circles it's much cooed over but I wouldn't take it, say, to Ascot. In the United States, the MoMA Design Store (81 Spring Street, New York 10012; 646-613-1367) sometimes has some Luisa Cevese pieces.

I have another seriously funky bag bought from the Contemporary Applied Arts shop at 2 Percy Street, London W1T 1DD; +44 20 7436 2344, which is made from a man's pinstriped suit fabric and the front is covered in buttons. It's by Edson Raupp, who seems to have a thing about buttons (or is it tailoring?), and I love it, most particularly because nobody ever knows where it's from. And it cost well under $400.

I nearly always have an Anya Hindmarch on the go. She does great totes; her bags look fashionable but don't shout, and for young mothers what could be nicer than her Photo Bag—a canvas tote with a picture of children and/or husband? Serious working women love her Bespoke Ebury, which you can order for some $1,500 from her own shop at 29 East Sixtieth Street, New York 10022; 212-750-3974.

For traveling I have a wonderful Meli-Melo, a great, soft carryall by Melissa del Bono (they're so soft that they pack flat, so you can take an extra one for bringing back the shopping), into which I can fit the requisite pashmina, book, change of shoes, toiletries, and other in-flight essentials.

For evening I have three favorites: a delicious little snake-skin number from Tanner Krolle with handles made of rough aquamarines; a small, very chic, plain black satin number with the frame edged in crystal and a slinky long handle by Judith Leiber of all people (she's mostly known for her exuber-antly glittery bags but she can do elegant very well when she wants to); and finally one of Ferragamo's brilliant little black beaded numbers.

Japanese designer Shizue (her shop, at 93 Mount Street, London W1K 2SY; +44 20 7491 3322, is a jewel in itself) is becoming something of a cult name sought out by those in the know on their trips to London. She creates little bag master-pieces. Some have a touch of the Japanese love of kitsch, others are over-the-top sumptuous, and yet others are just plain elegant. Almost all are like jewels, and if you add one to, say, a black evening outfit, it's as big and bold a statement as a brilliant necklace. If you haven't yet discovered Shizue, she's the de-signer who was the first to think of adding something as simple and practical as a light to her "opera" bag.

Another Japanese designer, Kazuyo Nakano (Cameron Diaz is said to be one of her fans), has ploughed a design fur-row of her own and though not quite as exotic as Shizue, nev-ertheless she comes up with fun and fashionable bags at pretty reasonable prices. Find her at 117 Crosby Street, New York 10012; 212-941-7093.

Cheaper Options

Chain stores these days are adept at copying the prevailing looks at extraordinarily good prices. In the U.K., Debenhams has some terrific bags at good prices and its designer collections—Jasper Conran's collection in particular—are always well worth looking out for. If you like the Birkin but can't afford its price tag, one of Jasper Conran's leather bags is a very good alternative, but most department stores have several good look-alikes. Furla is a very good middle-ranking brand to look out for—it has a knack of coming up with the currently fashionable shapes as well as some all-time classics. You could also look at the British label Jaeger, for instance, which has come up with some stunning bags that, while they're not cheap, are a whole lot better priced than the current "it" handbags from the fancier names. My own view is that if you can't afford leather, don't go for vinyl or plastic (unless it's really kitschy plastic, not plastic that is pretending to be leather); you're better to look for a fabric bag. I'm a fan of Accessorize, whose windows are a source of never-ending delight, filled as they are with brilliant colorways and intricate embroidery and beading. They always have a fantastic selection of inexpensive bags. And hang on to this fact: the divine Kate Middleton, Prince William's long-term fancy, looks a dream and is usually to be seen carrying nothing more pretentious than Longchamps and Bric's.

Bag Shoppers

Natalie Massenet, who runs net-a-porter.com, that compulsive site for the fashionaholic, has learned that there are three sorts of bag shoppers.

1. **The classic bag shopper**—the woman who goes for bags such as the Hermès Birkin bag. "This is the sort of bag that

looks right any time, any place, night or day. It's big, it's extravagant and it says loud and clear that you're rich, you're clever—and, most of all, you're lucky." It's the bag we buy ourselves when we've got a promotion, or have done a great deal, or it's the treat our husbands or partners buy for us if we're fortunate. The Chanel quilted 2.55 and Tomas Maier's Intrecito tote for Bottega Veneta will probably become new classics, as will most things by Marc Jacobs and Bottega Veneta.

And—a great tip—there's also the L. L. Bean tote bag, which Natalie Massenet calls "the Birkin of totes" ("It says you're rich and you're chic; you're just not quite so lucky"), which costs something like $20 and is an all-time classic. You can buy it online (www.llbean.com), and you can also get your name or initials embroidered on the bag for $6.

2. **The seasonal bag shopper**—the very smartly dressed woman who believes in having one or several new bags every season, all the very latest "must-haves" (probably most seasons this would mean a Chloé, a Prada, a Louis Vuitton, a Chanel, a Marc Jacobs, and a Mulberry), and then she sells them off in places like New York's La Boutique, Réciproque in Paris, or Sign of the Times in London when the season's over. Though how she could sell something as personal and intimate as a handbag is something of a mystery to the rest of us—as Natalie Massenet puts it, "I couldn't—it'd be like giving away a child."

3. The shopper who needs **a bag to suit every mood**—old, new, vintage, classic and wacky, practical and girly, funky and bold. Sharp girls around town who can't afford the latest "it" bag often opt for utilitarian bags such as satchels and messenger bags, which seem to say, "I've seen all the others but I chose something much more cool and street than anything "fashion-y."

A very good Massenet tip: "The young look great with something like a little Chanel handbag—the classic assurance of the Chanel bag is a good balance with funky youth.

It looks as if it's her first big treat, and it reads like a fashion statement. Contrarily, an older woman, I think, looks better with a cooler bag—it looks less staid. If she were to carry the Chanel bag it would seem more like a status symbol than a fashion statement. It's all about balance."

☞ *A really wacky present to give a friend who is besotted with her handbag is to organize a portrait of her handbag and its contents. Nathalie Lecroc (183 rue Saint Denis, 75002 Paris; +33 1 45 08 13 87) paints handbags and everything in them. She is most particular that her customers should be truthful and present their handbags as they are—not as they would like the world to think they are. Her watercolors are enchanting and she's surprisingly reasonable, charging something like $200.*

JEWELS

I love a bit of bling—not because it's expensive (which it needn't be) but for its decorative value. I don't have expensive heirloom pieces (sob, sob), because I didn't come from that sort of a family, though my mother gave me a very nice double string of pearls and my stepmother left me a wonderful diamond cluster ring for which I thank her daily. My husband has given me some lovely pieces but mostly of a rather contemporary nature, because he knows my tastes veer towards the funky and the quirky. I used to collect pretty bits of Victorian jewelry but I lost most of them in a burglary. Now I have one gorgeous string of gray-tinged South Sea pearls (bought from the divine Bob Reed of Linneys, 25 Dampier Terrace, Broome, Australia; www.linneys.com, and you should do the same if you're passing by), plus a couple of really good pairs of earrings. Otherwise it's mostly bits and bobs that I've collected since the burglary. My own favorite pieces include some amazing huge irregular blobs of red amber that I've already mentioned, which I bought in Oman, some great rough emeralds a friend found for me in

Colombia (I think), a necklace of rough turquoise, some Georgian amethyst earrings and a bracelet that is a coil of clear lime-green acrylic. In other words, I have eclectic tastes and most wardrobes need variety. Part of the point of all this is to say that while real can be wonderful (an amazing diamond or colored-stone piece from one of the great jewelers—who would say no?), it can also sometimes be quite staid and aging. Costume can be infinitely jollier, particularly when it comes to jewelry with attitude. A whole row of great bangles looks terrific—even cheap ones from markets in India, which cost literally pennies. Accessorize also does them brilliantly.

Jewelry used to be all about status and wealth but these days it is fundamentally there to be decorative, to light up the face, to enliven a sober outfit. An austere pantsuit can be given life if worn with some diamond studs in the ears for day and some glittery chandelier earrings for evening. Big cuffs are gorgeous, and fantastic brooches look great on jackets and dresses. But none of it has to be real. This winter I wore some glorious crystal and diamanté chandelier earrings that I bought from H & M for under $15 and several times had people compliment me on them and ask where I bought them.

Mlle Chanel was very addicted to her matching cuffs. They added glamour and pizzazz. These days cuffs are back in fashion. You could buy a whole wrist full of them at Claire's Accessories for under $30, while even most department stores sell big, bold cuffs and bracelets at very reasonable prices.

When traveling, a small wardrobe of some well-chosen costume jewelry means you can ring the changes with far fewer clothes. Come the evening, bring out the glitter—the dangling earrings, the fantastic necklace or the giant brooch. The trick, though, is not to pile it all on at once. A good rule, if you exclude wedding and engagement rings, is probably to stick to not more than two pieces at a time—earrings and a bracelet, a necklace and a bracelet, or earrings and a brooch. Just don't pile on the lot.

If you're doing costume jewelry though, don't do dinky. What's the point? It looks timid and uninteresting. Wear great chunky plastic discs or rough stones. A young girl I know has a wardrobe of huge swinging earrings that never fail to flatter and to catch the eye. If you ask her where she bought them, the answer is invariably Accessorize or Claire's Accessories. To buy—and wear—costume jewelry takes a bit more courage and something of an eye. You can't take refuge in the knowledge that it is by a grand designer but therein lies the fun.

Good Places to Buy

Barneys, 660 Madison Avenue, New York 10065, I scarcely need to tell you, has a fabulous jewelry collection—it's small, refined, carefully edited, and always exquisite.

Bergdorf Goodman, 754 Fifth Avenue, New York 10019—very sensibly—has jewelry that is just as desirable but offers an entirely different aesthetic from Barney's. It is less minimalist—it goes in for gorgeous chunks of rough stones and great big bracelets and gob-smackin' brooches—but it also always has a great collection of estate jewelry.

Ten Thousand Things, 423 West Fourteenth Street, New York 10014; 212-352-1333, is a tiny shop (but then jewelry doesn't take up a lot of room) that has lots of very contemporary pieces by up-and-coming designers such as David Rees and Lola Brooks.

Matter, 405 Broome Street, New York 10013; 212-343-2600; www.mattermatters.com, is mostly a furniture store selling avant-garde pieces (try the black skull candles) but there's also a collection of equally challenging jewelry by designers such as Nicole Landaw (said to be a Sarah Jessica Parker favorite—check out the spider brooch).

Boucher Jewelry, 9 Ninth Avenue, New York 10014; 212-206-3775, is a little gem of a shop with lots of semiprecious pieces that you could wear anywhere.

Deco Jewels, 131 Thompson Street, New York 10012; 212-253-1222, has great Lucite handbags and vintage costume jewelry that is high in decorative value and not so hard on the wallet.

Gas Bijoux, 238 Mott Street, New York 10012; 212-334-7290—terrifically fashionable beads and bracelets, much imported from France.

And never forget that these days many of the fashion brands—**Yves Saint Laurent, Marni, Chloé**—often provide eye-catching costume jewelry that is designed very specifically to complement their clothes. Marni's combination of cloth, beads, buttons and metal of a few years back were strangely beguiling and had nothing to do with the grand precious gems of yesteryear.

For weddings and engagements it has to be real, I think. Try the auction houses first (**Christie's, Sotheby's, Bonhams** and even the regional auction houses) for estate jewelry—the prices seem astonishingly good. Then there are some fabulous antique jewelry shops, of which my favorites in London have to be **Philips** at 139 New Bond Street, London W15 2TL; +44 20 7629 6261, and **Nigel Milne** at 38 Jermyn Street, London SW1Y 6DN; +44 20 7434 9343. But up and down the country there are good shops selling secondhand jewelry and the prices there are often surprisingly reasonable. Cheaper, and offering the additional thrill of a possible big "find," are places like **Greys Antique Market** in 58 Davies Street and 1–7 Davies Mews, London W1K 5AB; +44 20 7627 7034, or **Antiquarius** in the market at 131–141 King's Rd., London SW3 5EB.

Camden Passage in Islington (www.camdenpassageislington .co.uk) has lots of little antique shops worth exploring, not to mention its Saturday morning market where I've bought inexpensive silver, watches, and jewelry.

New York and most towns in America have great little shops that specialize in estate jewelry.

Doyle and Doyle at 189 Orchard Street, New York 10002; 212-677-9991, is many a New York fashionista's first stopping-off place for anything vintage or "antique" and not all of it costs a fortune—it has a good selection of engagement rings and pieces under $500. But look for great Art Deco brooches, Victorian rings, or Georgian earrings.

Young **James de Givenchy** (nephew of you-know-who) has been making a name for his jewels for some time now. He makes great vibrant one-off pieces, combining precious and semiprecious stones in the most gloriously insouciant way. He sees jewelry as "art." Every piece tells a story. Much sought-after by the charity-ball set. Find his wares at Taffin (685 Fifth Avenue, New York 10022; by appointment only, 212-421-6222).

Butler & Wilson, 189 Fulham Road, London SW3 6JN; +44 20 7376 5981, has fabulous costume jewelry, lots of bling and masses of funky brooches, necklaces and earrings.

Erickson Beamon, 38 Elizabeth Street, London SW1W 9NZ; +44 20 7259 0202, is a favorite with lots of fashionistas, selling pretty, delicate things at good prices.

Kiki McDonough, 77C Walton Street, London SW3 2HT; +44 20 7581 1777, has mastered the knack of giving the working woman the sort of jewelry that has just enough bling to give that frisson of pleasure and desire but not so much that it can't be worn in the boardroom. Droolingly desirable pieces in brilliant stones (she puts peridots with amethysts, for instance) at good prices.

Pippa Small (www.pippasmall.com) is the fashionista's current jeweler of choice, and I love her stuff, too. She takes rough stones and turns out huge interesting rings or asymmetrical lozenges of turquoise to form a necklace. Another necklace has a roughly cut diamond as a centerpiece. All fascinating. She has just opened her own shop at 11 Colville Mews, London W11 2DA. Also find her at The Cross, 141 Portland Road, London W11 4LR; +44 20 7727 6760, and at Kabiri, 37 Marylebone High Street, London W1U 4QE; +44 20 7224 1808 (a great jewelry shop, incidentally).

If it's just plain ol' diamonds that turn you on, you can buy them online in their pure and simple state and then get them set by a designer of your choice. www.abazias.com and www.bluenile.co.uk deliver both in the U.K. and the United States and offer lots of information as to the magic four Cs (cut, clarity, carat, and color) though these days many ask about the fifth C (conflict).

☛ *The theory behind buying diamonds in their simple state and online is that you get more diamond for your money because online retailing doesn't have the same overheads as retail shops.*

JEANS

I've come to the conclusion that it is really worth investing in a good pair of designer jeans. Provided your figure is in reasonable shape (and I don't mean you have to be a beanpole), it is amazing what a well-cut pair in a good, dark-washed denim can do. I now see why they're such a hit with the model set. Shoes are key—low pumps for a casual look, wedges for day and high heels for night make jeans wearable all day long. To solve the problem of the changing heel height, Radcliffe

Denim has come up with a brilliant (patented) solution in the shape of a cufflink that allows the wearer to change the length of the leg, lowering it for a stiletto, raising it for a pump. Older women, it goes without saying, shouldn't bare their midriffs. Wearing longer tops helps to make jeans look more grown-up as well as balance the lean silhouette below. Good jackets turn jeans into classy daywear. The wash is important—a dark, plain wash is the most sophisticated.

The semiotics of the premium jean are intricate and change almost daily. Tracking down that holy grail—a pair that makes one's behind look perkier, one's legs longer and one's stomach flatter—isn't easy so here are some places to get help.

The Perfect Jeans

The fad for the fancy-priced designer jean really arose on the West Coast, but a canny Brit, Suzy Radcliffe, took the notion and refined it even further. She made them less slouchy, less "West Coast" and much more urban and sophisticated. She called her brand Radcliffe Denim and it took off like a rocket. Here Suzy Radcliffe gives her guide to finding the perfect pair.

1. **Try on as many different brands and pairs as possible.** Find a store that has lots of different brands, grab every pair in your size (to start with) and try everything on. Don't even look at the brand name, just focus on finding the perfect pair.

2. **Try different sizes**—measurement differences are very subtle and vary according to the different denims and washes used. So if you think you are a size 28 waist, also try a 27 and a 29. Also try on two or three pairs of the same size as there will be minute differences between each pair, which may make one pair of size 28s fit better than another.

3. **Always think about comfort.** What you don't want is a pair of jeans that make you want to change out of them the

Where to Buy

Saks Fifth Avenue has "denim doctors" to help their jeans-obsessed customers orientate their way through the denim jungle.

If you're a jean aficionado you should try **Henry Lehr** at 9 Prince Street, New York 10012; 212-274-9921, where the staff are absolutely au fait with the semiotics of jean language. They'll know precisely which brands are the current cult name, what every brand says about its wearer, and guide you to the jean for you.

Jean Shop, 424 West Broadway, New York 10012; 212-334-5822, is the place where they'll tell you more about selvedges and the different sorts of denim that you might possibly want to know—but they'll also fit you with a great pair of jeans.

www.ilovejeans.com and **www.truejeans.com** (started by a man whose wife was reduced to tears because she couldn't find jeans that she really liked), two advisory Web sites that are a mine of useful information. Both guide you to the best jeans for your body shape.

minute you get home into something more comfortable. A great pair of jeans should not only look good but be as comfortable as your favorite pair of sweatpants. Key things to look out for are stretch denim (which will contour to your shape) and soft denim, i.e., that feels soft to the hand.

4. **Spend as much as you can** (or buy expensive jeans on sale). There is a reason why some jeans cost more than others. Premium brands will use expensive European and Japanese denims. They will also contain high-quality stretch fabrics that will retain their shape.

5. **Have different styles for different occasions**, don't just think, "I can only wear boot cut." Try trouser jeans, or a narrower pair with boots—this gives you a lot more wardrobe choices. Also try black and gray denim. Again, although you are still wearing jeans, the look is very different.

6. **There are styles suited to different body types.** As a general rule, boot cut (with a slight flare from the knee down) is universally the most flattering style. The boot cut balances out the hips and makes your legs look longer and slimmer. With narrower jeans (or skinny jeans) you need to think about boots and a heel but you don't need to be really skinny to wear these, especially if you team them with a long top or sweater.

T-Shirts

Most chains and mall stores have goodish versions, and it's hard to beat Gap and J. Crew for fit and price. I also love C & C California's T-shirts, which are brilliant and come in lots of colors. Otherwise look out for James Perse and Velvet labels, both of which have a great range of colors, with James Perse tending more towards the classic and Velvet towards the more fashionable shapes and colors. And remember, under the T-shirt you'll need a well-fitting seamless bra. Keep the lacy ones for another time.

Cashmere (. . . and How to Look After It)

One of my big new mantras is to adapt to the world of fashion that old Mies van der Rohe classic saying that was formulated for the domestic interior: "Less is more." I'd rather have fewer sweaters but most of them in cashmere than shelves full of lambswool. I work at home and my favorite working garment in the winter is a gorgeous gray cashmere sweater dress by Shirin Guild. It's my comfort blanket.

These days cashmere needn't be expensive—almost all mall shops and inexpensive chains sell it for ridiculously low prices, and mail-order companies such as Pure Collection (www.pure collection.com delivers to the United States) offer lots of classic cashmere lines. Which isn't to say that quality doesn't count—it does. The cheaper cashmere tends to fluff and ball far more than more expensive versions (it's usually made from the yarn from the back and the legs of the goat, which is coarser than that from the underbelly), whereas fine, expensive cashmere is not only made from the finest, white cashmere yarn but it is also properly treated and finished, which adds to the expense. Having spent all that money and loving on the garment itself, you don't want it to shrink or to be eaten away by moths. So here are my tips for looking after it.

You can wash it, if you dare. I have friends who wash it by hand; others put their cashmere in one of those laundry bags meant for delicate things and wash it on the delicates setting in their washing machines and it comes out looking terrific. I'd recommend using a special cashmere soap such as the Wool and Cashmere Shampoo from the Laundress (it is sulfate-free, comes in a choice of four scents and costs $18 from www.the laundress.com).

☞ *If you're nervous of washing cashmere yourself, check out the Laundress Web site (www.thelaundress.com), where the two girls who started the company give a riveting animated demonstration of how to wash cashmere. They also answer questions—very promptly—online.*

Belinda Robertson (+44 20 7838 9170; www.belinda robertson.com) does delicious cashmere that is always delivered in its own protection bag with a cedar block. But if you already own cashmere, and it didn't come in a bag, what do you do? First of all you get it properly cleaned. I would only ever use a really good laundry for this—my own in London happens to be Jeeves (www.jeevesofbelgravia.co.uk), which brings things back beautifully cleaned and wrapped, and they haven't shrunk a cashmere or a pashmina yet. Jeeves now has a branch at 39 East Sixty-fifth Street, New York 10065, but Montclair (1331 Lexington Avenue, New York 10128), Hallak Cleaners (1232 Second Avenue, New York 10065), as well as Madame Paulette (1255 Second Avenue, New York 10065) and Fashion Award Cleaners (2205 Broadway, New York 10024) all come highly recommended. And tucked away on almost every corner of most big cities are good laundry services (it's all those wonderfully hard-working immigrants). Belinda Robertson also offers a service that, for about $50 per garment, will wash and revive them (send to Belinda Robertson Edinburgh, 13A Dundas Street, Edinburgh EH3 6PG).

The price may seem high but it's better than losing your cashmere to moths. When you get your cashmere back from being cleaned, buy some plastic bags in which to store it (don't dream of doing this if you've already got moths—they'll have a field day inside the bag). Belinda Robertson will also sell you, at $5 each, the aromatic cedar blocks that promise to keep the moths at bay. I'm also told that putting cashmere in the freezer for at least twenty minutes is a good way of killing off all moths and their eggs.

If you already have moths and several holes (as I do in my beloved cashmere Shirin Guild sweater dress), do as Jeanetta Rowan-Hamilton of www.nettlescashmere.com does, and revive and customize the item by covering up the holes with charming pieces of old fabric edged with ribbon, embellished with buttons, stars, beads or lace.

Julia Dee, who runs a wardrobe care service (see also page 87), believes in storing cashmere in acid-free paper.

Specialist Help

Personal Shoppers and Wardrobe Advisors

I believe in them, not all the time (unless you're so rich or so busy that you pay one to do all your shopping for you) but to freshen up one's wardrobe. If you book a session with one of those on offer in most department stores (including, most excitingly, in the U.K., Topshop) they also cost nothing. You can just wave away anything you don't like and make them go on looking until they come up with something you do like. They look at one with a different eye and can, if they're good, wean one away from the safety of the tried and tested and give one a whole new look—or at least a few great new garments.

The big caveat is this: wardrobe advisors and personal shoppers are only as good as their advice. It sounds obvious, I know, but if you turn up for a personal shopping appointment (as I once did) and are met by a chap in the sort of suit you hoped never to see on a man you cared about, then you know you're not going to get the sort of advice you'd dream of taking. *But* when they're good, they're terrific. I've been given whole new looks and have been bought exciting garments that I'd never have thought of through good advisors but it's absolutely key to make sure your taste meshes with his/hers.

Ones who've worked for me are Celia Clarke at Liberty (Regent St., London W1B 5AH)—she found for me a fabulous Missoni coat that cost a bomb but has earned its keep time and time again, as well as a grass-green Armani jacket that is to die for and that I'd never have dared to pick out on my own, as well as a brilliant grayish/blackish/brownish cloque evening jacket by the Turkish designer Ischiko. Martina Wagener at Selfridges (400 Oxford Street, London W1A 1AB) found for me my favorite skirt in the world—a black Ischiko one with huge black silk roses in a cluster on one side—as well as a brilliant steel gray satiny Marni coat with bracelet sleeves and a little stand-up collar that will look good for the rest of my life. *Very* Audrey Hepburn. All this advice came free—though the bill for the clothes was another matter. However, I console myself with the thought that I love the things I bought and I know I wouldn't have found them on my own.

Of course the personal shopper was invented in the U.S. and it's no surprise to find that almost all good stores have terrific personal shoppers—and the service they offer is efficient, personal, and, if you have the funds (it's really not worth going if you only have peanuts to spend) can transform the way you dress. Take Elaine Mack, Bergdorf's star personal shopper. She helped invent the genre way back when there was a Bergdorf's out in Westchester where the Goodmans themselves lived. For her favored clients she looks out for the blouse that will go with the skirt you've already got, the jacket that gives double life to the pants, the just so tights . . . and so on and on. Her clients get little phone calls telling them what's just arrived, what's hot, what will suit them and then, if they bite, it all gets couriered over to them—whether they live in San Francisco, Chicago, or around the corner. She gets very booked up so you should book an appointment at 212-872-8810.

At Barney's many a socialite goes to Sharyn Soleimani (ssoleimani@barneys.com).

There are lots of personal shoppers who will come to the house, look through your wardrobe, tell you what to keep and what to throw away. Then they will hold you by the hand and take you shopping to fill in the gaps and freshen the whole lot up. If they're any good, they will know the merchandise in a whole host of shops, have good relationships with many of them and so can arrange to have things put aside, and often they can get you to private sample sales and previews. This kind of service can be wonderful but it isn't usually cheap. And remember the big caveat: they are only as good as their taste.

The best way to find a good one is by asking friends.

Here are a few I can recommend.

IN THE UNITED STATES

There are, of course, the stylists to the stars—**Phillip Bloch** in San Francisco (323-874-4979; www.phillipbloch.com) who's credited with looking after Sandra Bullock, Salma Hayek, and lots of other stars of stage and screen, and **Rachel Zoe** (Nicole Richie, Lindsay Lohan, Jessica Simpson) to name but two—and wonderful though they may be I think those of us who lead more earth-bound lives might find we didn't get their full and undivided attention.

Amanda Ross, a gorgeous ex-magazine stylist, used to work at *Harper's Bazaar* and now works on a freelance basis helping to put together the wardrobes of anybody who needs help. She charges $3,000 a day. Contact her on www.amandaross.com.

Stacey Mayesh used to be a senior fashion editor at *Marie Claire*—these days she'll come to your home, sort your wardrobe, and help find a style that's right for you. Contact her via www.staceymayesh.com. She charges $350 an hour.

Jesse Garza and Jo Lupo (212-315-2233; www.visual-therapy.com) work as a team and come with impressive credentials (they work for Bergdorfs and Ian Schrager, as well as private individuals)—they'll do anything from finding something for the red carpet to turning out your wardrobe and advising what to keep and what to throw. They work in Chicago, New York, and the West Coast.

Eric Launder, 2 Gold Street, New York 10038; 917-769-8978, is said by those in the know (most particularly by Grant Thatcher, founder and editor in chief of the *Luxe Guides*) to be one of New York's best personal stylists with what he calls a "mind boggling knowledge of the city's stores."

Literary agent Linda Chester swears by **Rig Maxfield**, 225 East Fifty-seventh Street, Apt. 19D, New York 10022 (redman maxfield@mac.com; 212-751-9292), who is responsible for many a high society woman's glossy look.

IN THE U.K.

Amanda Platt (+44 20 7229 8109) is style guru to legions of Notting Hill yummy mummies as well as to elegant middle-aged professionals, tycoons' wives and others far too famous to tell on. More to the point, she's also used to dealing with those of us who aren't as young, tall, blonde, or fashion savvy as we'd like. She's also *very* nice: none of this "My God, where did you find that skirt?" line, which would have most of us cowering in a corner in no time at all. You can safely go to her with the frumpiest of wardrobes and she'll have you organized in two shakes. She costs $1,100 a day, and for that she will sort out your wardrobe, tell you what is hot and great in the shops at the moment, take you shopping or just make a list of things she thinks you should buy. She has fabulous taste and really knows her shops and her brands. She also gets very booked up.

Camilla Yonge of Y Shop (+44 7711 277 969 and at www.y-shop.co.uk) is young, nice, energetic, and knows her stock. She'll come to the house, suss your style, and then find you stuff that you'd never have found by yourself.

Leesa Whisker (+44 870 043 4126 and at www.whisker agency.co.uk) is rumored to be the style consultant behind Kate

Middleton's very ladylike look, which is—when you think about it—perfect for the role she has to play. People who've tried Leesa Whisker tell me she's terrific with a great sense of style. She isn't cheap but almost everybody who's used her says it was great value. She costs $600 for a home visit and $800 for a full shopping day.

Jo Poole (aka The Dress Doctor, +44 7855 032 705 and at www.thedressdoctor.co.uk) is a costumier at the National Theatre and also works for the BBC. She runs a wonderful mobile fitting and alteration service. She'll come, look at your wardrobe, and tell you what's worth keeping and what's not. Furthermore, she will alter and—get this—drastically remake something that you love but that no longer quite works. She costs about $300 for a day's worth of advice and my young colleague at *The Times,* Alice Olins, swears by her.

www.dressme.biz (+44 7734 870 567) will do as much or as little as you'd like. Somebody will come to the house, sort your wardrobe, tell you what they think works and what doesn't, what you should wear with what, and show you how to make the most of the things you already have. They can restyle, reorganize, and either go shopping for you or take you shopping. You choose.

Shona Mac (+44 20 7349 7225 and at www.shonamac .com) charges about $100 an hour for which she'll come to the house, go through your wardrobe, tell you what to keep, what to throw out and—even better—she'll help you sell the discarded clothes (on eBay) and, obviously for a fee, revitalize and update clothes worth saving. The classic rule for wardrobe sorting always used to be "If you haven't worn it for two years, throw it out." I'm not much of a believer in that since I'm currently wearing things that have lain dormant for much longer than that. So an experienced second eye from somebody like Shona Mac is, in my view, well worth having.

How to Get Rid of Unwanted Clothes

Since most fashion writers would have one believe that in order to hold one's head up in what passes for society, one needs to be carrying the latest bag, wearing the hot shoe and be clad in something seen not so long ago on the catwalk, it follows that those who adopt this advice will either have to live in a mansion or else colonize whole rooms that should ideally be used for purposes other than storing clothes. In my opinion the only answer to wardrobe chaos is regularly to edit the contents. I'm not much good at this myself and have been known to search desperately for the right skirt/jacket/shirt for an unconscionable amount of time simply because the wardrobe is too full or too chaotic.

The golden mantra when contemplating, say, a new pair of cropped pants, has to be: ask yourself firmly, (a) do I need it? (b) is it better than its close relation already in the wardrobe? and (c) when will I will wear it? Only if you have satisfactory answers to all three should you buy it. *Then* you must make up your mind to throw out its earlier, less useful/attractive counterpart.

If you have designer gear to sell, eBay is the current favorite of choice if you can manage the technology—taking the photograph, signing up, and then posting it on the site. If you can't, there is www.ebay-kit-free.com, a company that sells kits designed to take the hassle out of the matter. It tells you exactly how to manage the whole process. iSold It (www.i-soldit.com) has a chain of stores across the country where you can just drop your no-longer-wanted goods and they do all the rest—for a commission (somewhere between 33 and 40 percent, depending upon the item) of course, whereas if you can do it yourself on eBay you keep the lot.

Some personal shoppers will—for a fee—obviously do all this for you, including Shona Mac (see page 85).

Never forget the charity shops—your unwanted sweaters could be literally a lifesaver for somebody in the poverty-stricken areas of the world. Speaking personally, as I travel a great deal, I always take a bag full of cast-offs if I'm heading off to remote regions in Africa or India.

Cleaning, Alterations, Repairs, and Storage

Dynasty Custom Tailors at 6 East Thirty-eighth Street, New York 10016; 212-679-1075, are the alterations experts the voguettes swear by (ask for Joe).

Julia Dee of Designer Alterations (220A Queenstown Road, London SW8 4LP; +44 20 7498 4360 and at www .designeralterations.com)—or one of her team—will come and sort out your wardrobe. They'll mend, clean, repair and—a huge boon for those who live in small spaces—they'll store your off-season clothes, thus allowing you to have a wardrobe twice the size. The perfumer Jo Malone, who lived in a small flat in her earlier days, told me that Julia Dee enabled her then to have a decent wardrobe. Jo kept each season's clothes at home and when the season was over she got Julia Dee to collect, clean, wash, repair and stow them away. At the same time Julia would bring the new season's clothes out of storage, all fresh and ready to wear.

Linda Agran (+44 845 083 0111 and at www.linda agran.co.uk, or e-mail info@lindaagran.co.uk) offers much the same service but at the Rolls-Royce end. Clothes are collected, mended, cleaned, and otherwise restored to their pristine state. The ones you don't need are stored in "a precisely controlled environment" until you need them again. Clients get little albums, with digital photographs of all their garments, so that they can remember what it is they actually own and summon it for the right occasion. When they need an item, they either call or check-in online and the garment can be returned at a couple

Storage and Stuff

These are great companies for good hangers, acid-free paper, and proper storage containers for clothes.

UNITED STATES

Gracious Homes, which has four branches in New York (one on the West Side and three on the East Side) and now sells its wares online (www.gracious homes.com), is a much underrated source of all the small practical aids one needs to keep a house or apartment in good running order. It sells canvas and plastic storage of every kind, the just-right hangers and, besides, its Web site is a fund of truly useful advice.

Closet Organizers USA (www.closetorganizersusa .com) and **The Container Store** (www.container store.com) both sell online all the small accessories that help keep a closet in good order.

U.K.

Lakeland (www.lakeland.co.uk) is a great British gem—and it ships to the United States so work your fingers to get a catalog now. It sells all those incredibly useful things that we all need to make our lives tick and in particular it has everything you need to keep the moths at bay as well as wardrobe organizers and transparent (so you can check the contents) boxes to store shoes or sweaters.

The Holding Company (call +44 20 8445 2888 for a catalog), started in the U.K. by Dawna Walter, an American deeply shocked at the state of the average British closet, who developed a mission to put them in order, has all manner of storage suggestions, including trays to help keep socks, tights and small items in order, plus an array of products to ward off moths. It will also ship to the U.S.

of hours' notice if need be. However, you can't stow away just the odd sweater. There's a minimum charge of $600 worth of storage per quarter *but* that includes one free collection and delivery. Express delivery is extra—$100.

Garde Robe (www.garderobeonline.com and 212-227-7554) does all that for New Yorkers. It will collect, clean and repair your garments, photograph and catalog them and then—if you need it—they'll store it all in a climate-controlled, air-purified loft. If you're handy with the mouse you can manage it all—delivery, collection, storage—online.

THE SALES

I'm not a big fan of them: the pushing, the shoving, the ugly faces, and the even uglier fracas. On the whole I'd rather do without than face the sheer awfulness of it all. Which isn't to say that you shouldn't always peruse the sales rails during normal, calmer times—many a bargain has been uncovered there. However, there are some things really well worth buying in sales and they're usually still there after the first hectic days are over. If you're either very small or very tall, there are fantastic bargains to be had in the clothes and shoe lines. Clothes apart, lots of fine staples are always reduced: stationery, soap, luggage, linen, and electronics, not to mention things like washing machines and dishwashers with the odd immaterial scratch.

There are of course two great classic places to find great bargains—New York's Century 21 (22 Cortland Street, New York 10007; www.c21stores.com) and Boston's Filene's Basement (497 Boylston Street, Boston 02116; www.filenesbasement .com). Both of them require huge reserves of energy and you need to be prepared to devote considerable time to the project

but you can come away with terrific bargains of every kind—
from Ralph Lauren sheets to the perfect cashmere.

Here are my golden rules for clothes shopping in the sales:

1. Only buy something you really love or actually need.

2. Buy the bit of magic you couldn't otherwise afford.

3. If it doesn't fit in the shop, that won't change by the time
   you get it home.

4. Never buy anything too small. Only buy something too
   large if you have a crackingly good tailor.

5. Avoid the boring classics—it's better to buy them in your
   own good time in a solid high street shop where there is no
   danger of being panicked into a buy—and where you know
   you can always take things back.

6. Keep away from anything in a bin or with "special purchase" attached to it.

7. If there's something you've really set your heart on and you
   know it's going to be reduced, then plan your venture like a
   military recce. Scout out the joint first and then plot the
   quickest route to your quarry.

8. Don't be tempted to buy something in a wild color that
   you'd never wear simply because it's 50 percent off.

9. If you're liable to be tempted, take a good and honest friend
   with you—if she says don't do it, then listen up.

10. Before you part with your hard-earned cash, check the
    shop's refund policy.

TWO

how

to

look

good

Why It Matters

I'm not—and never have been—a specialist beauty writer, but I'm awfully keen on looking as good as I can. I've also written and edited what these days are called "lifestyle pages" in newspapers for more years than I'm going to tell you about here, and beauty has always been part of my beat. So though I'm not an expert I've been inundated (oh, bliss) with goodies from efficient publicists getting me to test their wares. I've tried a lot of things, met an awful lot of "experts," visited countless labs and interviewed more purveyors of lotions and potions than I can possibly count. I've been swathed in oils in India, stood on my head in Bali, been hosed down in Arizona, wrapped in hot towels in Paris, had sound therapy with gongs in Africa and lots, lots more. I wish I could say with certainty that I always know what works and what doesn't, but to be truthful, I can't always tell. Some things you just *know* work for you, and even if they don't, they're so enjoyable that you don't much care. Others you may have a hunch are doing their job and others may leave you mystified.

The beauty business isn't an exact science. You can never be sure how you would have looked if you hadn't tried a specific cream/regime/treatment. When the rather cynical men on the newspaper for which I worked used to imply that the whole beauty industry was bunkum, merely a way of generating huge sums for their manufacturers, I always had the same reply: "I can't give you rational, scientific proof, but just look around you. The evidence is there. Those who take trouble look a whole lot better than those who don't." I certainly know that I look better for taking the best care of my skin that I can, and as for wearing makeup, speaking personally, I do not step outside without it, even to go to the supermarket.

So I'm of the opinion that it's worth taking some care of yourself—both the inner and the outer being. It was George Burns who famously remarked: "If I'd known I was going to live this long, I'd have taken better care of myself." Well, many of us—praise be—are going to live much longer than our forebears so we might as well make it as enjoyable as possible. Being fit and healthy, and looking as good as we can, seem to me an essential component of the good life. Apart from anything else, healthy, good-looking people add to the gaiety of the nation—it's a form of politeness to others. Being unfit and overweight, short of breath or—worse—unable to walk unaided—isn't fun. Although some ill health is not always avoidable, if we try to eat the right things and stay away from the bad ones most of the time, if we take a modicum of exercise and keep an eye on the warning signs (high blood pressure, high cholesterol, obesity), then we are at least giving our bodies more of a chance to last the course without disaster overtaking us. As an eminent doctor put it on the news recently: "We probably can't extend people's lifespan much longer than we already have, so our efforts now are concentrated on trying to enable people to be as healthy as possible for as much of that lifespan as possible."

I don't believe in being obsessive (there's nothing so unattractive and miserable as women who won't eat a thing after five P.M.—or who toy with a few lettuce leaves while everyone else longs for a decent glass of wine) but I do believe that light, delicious food that goes easy on the fat and sugar is not only healthier than junk food but makes you feel better and more alive. I also know that moderate exercise is hugely enjoyable (at least it is for me; there's nothing I like better than being on a ski slope or a tennis court, though jogging bores me to tears) and it keeps the muscles firm, the heart in good shape, and the mind alert.

But you shouldn't confuse looking good with trying to look younger than you are—they're not the same thing at all. The French seem to understand that better than we do and while you see older French women who are enormously chic, as a rule they seldom look ridiculous. Women who take a modicum of trouble can look good at any age without trying to pass themselves off as anything that they are not. On the other hand I don't think trying *too* hard is attractive, either. It speaks of narcissism and vanity, of a lack of proportion in one's life and of other, proper interests. We've all seen those examples of Tom Wolfe's famous social X-ray skeletons, whose over-made-up elderly faces and frail figures look quite scary. The aim surely should be to try to get the balance right, to work out what suits you and what doesn't, and then to get on with the more interesting parts of life.

Nevertheless there are lots of wonderful treatments available that really do make a difference—not just to how you look but, perhaps more importantly, to how you feel. After I was mugged some years ago, which left my mouth lopsided and out of kilter, two plastic surgeons—Howard Sobel in New York and Barry Jones in London—between them kindly put the whole thing right, and the difference it has made to my morale is huge. My smile will never be quite what it was but at least now I show the same amount of teeth on both sides when I smile. So I'm a fan of plastic surgery (more about this later). I'm also a fan of treatments that work. I've had letters from women who were almost in tears of joy at the uplift to their spirits when their broken veins, brown spots, under-eye bags and crepey décolletages were attended to. They weren't excessively vain; rather they were understandably mourning the loss of their youthful skin and looks, and the discovery that some of the damage could be repaired restored their self-esteem no end.

☞ *Like many, I am a great fan of* Feel Fabulous Forever *by Josephine Fairley and Sarah Stacey; their latest news is always worth checking out on www.beautybible.com.*

I'm not attempting here to give you a rundown on the complete beauty market place—whole tomes would be needed for that alone. I'm passing on only what I've learned over the years and mentioning only therapies or products that have really worked for me and my friends.

I'm tired of all this business of beauty being only skin deep.
That's deep enough. What do you want—an adorable pancreas?
—JEAN KERR, WRITER

SKIN

I'm starting here because it matters most. With naturally gorgeous skin, you can get away with almost no makeup but my advice is, don't take it for granted. Do all you can to make sure it stays as good as it can. The key to good skin is keeping out of the sun, eating well, drinking lots of water (while keeping off tea, coffee, and alcohol if you can; I personally can't do without small amounts of all three!) and then following the three mantras of cleanse, tone, nourish. And these days we have to add exfoliating to the list. Exfoliating gets rid of the dead cells; our skins shed them at a fantastic rate each day—though more slowly as we get older—and if they accumulate they make the skin look dull. Remove them and the skin instantly (and I really mean instantly) looks more radiant. And one more thing: if you care about your skin, you shouldn't go near a cigarette—ever.

If you have a few brown spots, broken capillaries or other imperfections, remember that today there are brilliant ways of dealing with them. IPL lasers deal beautifully with both red veins and brown spots. Almost all good dermatologists and aestheticians now have access to these lasers so there's no need to suffer in silence.

Cleansers

I don't think soap and water cuts it. I've tried it, but it leaves my skin feeling harsh and dry. However, if you're hard up, I don't think that it makes sense to buy an expensive cleanser. Even the simplest—e.g., Liz Earle (from QVC), L'Oreal, and Boots (which is available at Target stores and the Body Shop)—do a really good job. If your budget allows it, here are a few of my favorites.

Shu Uemura's Cleansing Oil appears at first to be very oily, but as soon as it hits the skin it turns milky, removing every scrap of makeup while at the same time leaving the skin feeling as if it has been nourished as well as cleansed. Clever old Mr. Uemura got the idea for it way back in the 1960s when he was making up the stars in Hollywood. He observed that Marilyn Monroe, Liz Taylor, and Shirley MacLaine (not to mention—though whisper it quietly—Frank Sinatra) all had to resort to oil to remove the heavy makeup needed for the cameras. He therefore set about refining oil to make it more user-friendly. The current cleansing oil—and there are many versions, devised to cope with every skin type—is made from olive oil, sunflower oil, jojoba oil, and a couple of other secret ingredients.

Guerlain has some brilliant new cleansing products called Secret de Pûreté. They contain lotus flower (which is claimed to be known for its purity and its restorative properties) but, more to the point, they leave the skin feeling divine. There are creams, milks, foams, and gels. I recommend the Eye and Lip Makeup Remover. (You need to be particularly careful about what you use to remove eye makeup—I only ever use a cleanser specifically meant for eyes.) I like the texture of Guerlain's milky cleanser best.

Liz Earle's Naturally Active Cleanse and Polish Hot Cloth Cleanser (it comes as a little bottle plus two muslin cloths) is wonderful and not expensive, about $24.50 (www .lizearle.com).

Eve Lom's cleanser, which lots of women I respect swear by, also comes with little muslin cloths. It's a cult product that many are addicted to. Find it at Space NK (www.spacenk.com).

Exfoliators

There's a bit of controversy over these in that some women think they're a bit harsh on the skin. As I've already pointed out earlier, exfoliators remove dead cells that can clog the pores and prevent the skin looking its best. I'm a believer. Deep cleansing and exfoliating are partly the point of a facial and I notice that my skin always looks infinitely more radiant afterwards. I don't use them every day; once a week is just right for me. If you're prone to broken veins and have very sensitive skin, go carefully and use only the gentlest versions. My skin can't take anything harsh, so I like Liz Earle's Naturally Active Gentle Face Exfoliator, but there are lots on the market at every price range.

You can also buy exfoliators in pad form—particularly useful when traveling; you simply use one a day—or as lotions or creams. At the cheaper end, Origins Modern Friction is, with good reason, a cult product, and Valentine Alexander (my makeup guru, who tries almost everything that comes on the market) tells me that Olay's Definity Pore Redefining Scrub is brilliant. At the more luxurious end of the market, Givenchy's Black Mask is good while Dr. Hauschka's Rejuvenating Mask makes the skin look more radiant. Take your pick. If it suits your skin, stick with it. If it leaves it red and irritated, try something else.

Toners

I'm not too fussy here and wouldn't think it worth going for a high-cost toner. Just make sure to choose one that isn't too astringent and is alcohol-free.

Moisturizers

It depends on your skin type which one is for you—dry skins and older skin need richer moisturizers than oily skin and young skin—but absolutely key is to make sure it has an SPF of at least 15 (preferably more) and that you wear it every day. In your twenties that's probably all you need but the older you get, the more you should ask of your moisturizer. Look for hydrating properties in your thirties, antiaging ones in your forties and, after that, choose ultrarich, deeply moisturizing versions. They'll cost more but here spending a bit more really buys extra benefits. If you have good skin with an even skin tone, you may be able to get away with just wearing a tinted moisturizer that matches your skin color.

Nourishing Creams

You can spend peanuts (on something like Nivea, Vaseline, or Neutrogena), or you can spend, literally, hundreds of dollars. I think nourishing creams make a big difference, particularly as you get older. Those targeted at aging skin have active ingredients that help cell renewal (the main reason for skin beginning to look dingy is that the rate of cell renewal decreases greatly with age). They also boost collagen production, plump up the skin, and penetrate deeper into the epidermis.

I don't think there are such things as miracle creams but I am absolutely convinced that regularly nourishing the skin keeps it softer, plumper and slows down the rate at which wrinkles develop. I do *not* think that the whole beauty industry is one big con—serious research goes into these creams and cutting-edge ingredients cost more than run-of-the-mill ones. I would no more dream of going to bed at night without using a night cream than I would miss cleaning my teeth.

If you want real proof of what good creams can do, a few brands (the Japanese company SK-II for one, DCL or Dermatologic Cosmetic Laboratories, and Elemis) use high-tech Visia Medical Imaging Systems to photograph the skin before and after treatment in order to track the changes in wrinkles, skin texture, brown spots, et al.

It's almost impossible to single out one cream from among all the others, for what suits one person's skin doesn't suit someone else's. *But* the problem is that trying out all of them is an expensive business—who wants to spend $400 on something and then find it doesn't suit their skin? The best advice I can offer is to suggest you consult Josephine Fairley and Sarah Stacey's *Feel Fabulous Forever* (published by Penguin, $35), in particular the chapter titled "Tried and Tested Miracle Creams," the result of a trial of some sixteen hundred women aged thirty-five or more.

Some inexpensive products work brilliantly well—Boots has a product called No. 7 Protect and Perfect Beauty Serum in the U.K., but it is also sold in U.S. outlets (mostly at Target, www.target.com) under the name No. 7 Restore and Renew Beauty Serum for $21.99. It's chiefly worth mentioning because in a recent television show that looked seriously at the matter of skin care, it came out as the topmost performing antiaging cream. Sales soared by some 2,000 percent. But it is worth bearing in mind that the more expensive houses—Estée Lauder, Guerlain, Sisley, La Prairie—may appear from the labels to use the same ingredients as cheaper makes, but there are cheap liposomes and expensive liposomes, cheap essential oils and expensive ones, and the grander names do, usually, use better ingredients. Also you don't need to slather the stuff on. Use it sparingly. The younger you are, the less you need to have of these age-defying creams.

Here are some of my own favorites:

Chantecaille's Biodynamic Lifting Cream isn't cheap (about $295 a pot) but it has a cult following. It is stuffed full of natural ingredients but they have been carefully researched and have a proven effect. One of the key ingredients (the one that has elicited the "liquid Botox" quip) is hexapeptide, which interferes with the messages that tell muscles to contract and therefore inhibits frowning and lines. Another, tocotrienols, which are said to be some fifty times more potent than Vitamin E, help fight free radicals and protect collagen elasticity. There are also lots of lovely, delicious essential oils—magnolia, rose, and many more.

Guerlain's Issima line is one that I love, in particular its Midnight Secret—it feels richly nourishing and yet not heavy.

Natura Bissé's Diamond Extreme Cream is a current favorite with me (as it is, apparently, with Sienna Miller, Naomi Campbell, and Keira Knightley) but it is phenomenally expensive (about $300 a pot, from Neiman's). I love both its texture and its delicious, slightly herby smell, although it's too expensive to use all the time so I'll move to something less expensive when this pot is finished.

Sisley Global Anti-Age is another expensive one (nearly $450), but brilliantly rehydrating and nourishing.

Estée Lauder's Re-Nutriv Ultimate Lifting Crème is another enormously expensive cream but it has a whole cocktail of active antiaging ingredients and it feels very good to use.

Lancôme's Nutrix Royal is not too expensive (something like $50) and is a long-time favorite of many mature women so it must have something going for it.

SK-II's Facial Treatment Essence is a cult cream in Japan. It contains 90 percent pitera, an ingredient discovered by a Japanese monk visiting a sake brewery in Kobe who happened to notice that elderly workers there had extraordinarily soft, young-looking hands. He embarked on five years experimentation, during which he eventually discovered that pitera, a nutrient-rich by-product of yeast fermentation, contained a collection of vitamins, minerals, amino, and organic acids that had a remarkable effect on the skin. SK-II's Facial Treatment Essence was the result. It has remained unchanged in formula—and in price (at the time deemed astronomical) since it was launched just over twenty years ago.

Crème de la Mer is enormously expensive and, confusingly, it is referred to as a moisturizer but in fact it really does the job of a nourishing cream. Many women swear by it. Its formula has a serious basis. Years ago, aerospace physicist Dr. Max Huber suffered a horrific accident—a routine experiment exploded in his face—which gave him severe chemical burns. Neither science nor medicine offered much promise of help, so Huber decided to help himself. Twelve years and six thousand experiments later, he perfected the cream that would help give skin a dramatically smoother appearance.

At the heart of this cream is a highly potent Miracle Broth. There is nothing miraculous about its ingredients—sea kelp, calcium, magnesium, potassium, iron, lecithin, vitamins C, E, and B_{12}, plus oils of citrus, eucalyptus, wheat germ, alfalfa, and sunflower. For Huber, it wasn't the ingredients but the way those ingredients were distilled that made all the difference between a good moisturizer and a small miracle. No doubt Huber understood the ancient science of biofermentation. He discovered that as these ingredients changed from individual components into a rich Miracle Broth (a process that took three or four months to complete), they did indeed transform into a whole far greater than the sum of its parts.

At the less expensive end of the spectrum, apart from **Boots' No. 7 Restore and Renew Beauty Serum**, which is a star product, there is **Neal's Yard Remedies Frankincense Nourishing Cream**, costing something like $35.

Sarah Stacey, beauty editor and coauthor (with Jo Fairley) of *The Beauty Bible* and *Feel Fabulous Forever,* reveals her own favorite nighttime miracle workers. She recommends that you apply them all with gentle upward strokes from neck/décolletage to hairline. And, she says, around the eye bone you should merely tap the cream in.

FOR DAILY USE IN SUMMER, OR ALL YEAR ROUND
Balm Balm Rose Geranium Organic Face Balm
(just $12 from www.beautyhabit.com).
This is a fantastic value, heavenly smelling, totally organic balm that works on skin anywhere, as well as tames flyaway hair. My desert-island must-have. Brilliant at night, or for daytime if you're not using a matte antishine foundation because it takes a wee bit of time to sink in, with the result that you look shiny and your base can slip off, but it's fine under tinted moisturizer.

FOR EXTRA HELP IN WINTER
Aromatherapy Associates Renew Rose & Frankincense Facial Oil ($44 from www.spacenk.com).

(continues)

(continued)
Again, there is a lift-your-spirits fragrance in this oil from a leading aromatherapy company. Rose and frankincense essential oils are legendary for soothing, repairing, and reinvigorating skin. You need only a couple of drops, so it lasts nearly for ever.

TO SOUP UP TIRED, BLAH SKIN

Dr. Bragi Age Management Marine Enzyme, ($240 for a 1.7-ounce dispenser, from Bliss).

This is hugely expensive but you need to use just one or two pumps per application. I keep it for when my skin really looks in need of help. This marine-based "penzyme" (penetrating enzyme) was developed by a leading professor of biochemistry at the University of Iceland as a treatment for wound healing and arthritis. Its light gel formulation is truly antiaging, making skin amazingly smoother, tauter, and brighter, in my experience. And stacks of testimonials attest that it is effective, too, for problem skin conditions including acne, rosacea, and eczema. Dr. Bragi also says it will help scarring and dark circles.

The War Against Wrinkles

In your twenties: Wear sunscreen and, when out in the sun, a sunhat as well. The skin can still repair itself but light exfoliating with an alpha-hydroxy acid product will remove dead skin and give the skin a smoother look.

In your thirties: Greater nourishment is needed and retinol products will help plump up fine lines. If your skin starts to look dry, use a really good moisturizer.

In your forties: Look for richer nourishing creams with antiaging properties (suitable creams and lotions will all carry this label). Some therapists recommend very light, glycolic acid-based peels once a month to reduce fine lines and facial brown spots or uneven skin tone.

In your fifties and over: You should be using products specifically labeled antiaging or one of the cult creams referred to above. Creams containing retinol have been proven to improve the look of wrinkles by boosting the production of key skin-building compounds such as glycosaminoglycan and collagen. You might like to consider the newer serums, which generally contain cocktails of antioxidants and alpha-hydroxy acids, and should be worn under your usual moisturizer. Many women swear by them. Particularly recommended is Cellex-C High Potency Serum, and I also very much like Origins Mega-Mushroom Face Serum, especially around the eye area, where they are less irritating than rich nourishing creams.

I have seen photographic evidence of amazing results from chemical peels, dermabrasion, laser resurfacing, and microdermabrasion—with deep wrinkles almost eliminated and the skin looking completely refreshed—*but* they should be applied only by a proper dermatologist who can assess whether these procedures will work for you. Some can leave the skin very sensitive and red for weeks. Most dermatologists now recommend a series of mild peels rather than one really deep, medical peel.

Remember that some wrinkles are not only inevitable but not necessarily unattractive. Older faces where all lines have been eliminated by face-lifts, Botox, and their ilk look curiously unlived-in.

Treats and Facials

I'm a believer in facials. I don't go in for them very often (time and money, those perennial twin bugbears) but when the skin is tired and jaded a good one undoubtedly gets rid of all the old, dead skin, massages the skin so that it is more oxygenated and the oils, masks or lotions leave it much more hydrated. The net result is skin that is noticeably livelier and more radiant.

Tracie Martyn gives the kind of facials that used to have several of Manhattan's glossy set making pilgrimages across the Brooklyn Bridge—but lucky for them the dear lambs don't have to do that any more because Tracie Martyn now has her salon in Manhattan itself in the more salubrious surrounds of 59 Fifth Avenue, New York 10003; 212-206-9333. She's most famous for her Resculpting Facials, which many of her actor/actress clients have just before the Oscars—it's said to do non-surgically what otherwise only the knife will do. She uses a particular combination of massage, electric current (which she channels through her own Resculptor machine) *and* her custom-made creams to tighten muscles in ways that would, say her fans, take months of exercise to achieve.

Others these days go to her for "a better bottom"—yes, really. She now has a Resculptor machine adapted for the body and all its sagging ills—those who have tried it swear it attacks cellulite and reshapes the body. Kate Winslet and Susan Sarandon are both said to be fans. Well, there's not a lot to lose, except a wad of dollars.

Wendy Lewis, dubbed "the Knife Coach" for her impartial advice on the best aesthetic treatments, says her favorite facialist in New York is **Denise DeGiulio** at Enhanced Image, 130 West Fifty-seventh Street, New York 10019; 212-957-0777—she gives a medical-grade facial and peelings and is very experienced in all manner of cosmetic treatments. Down in Soho **Dr. Laurie Polis's spa** (62 Crosby Street, New York 10012; 212-431-1600; www.mezzaninespa.com) is much frequented by the high maintenance set. Wendy's richer clients also love Katia at **Anushka Spa, Salon & Cosmedical Centre** in Palm Beach

(701 South Rosemary Avenue, West Palm Beach 33401; 561-820-0500; www.anushkaspa.com).

Tracey Ross, who owns the legendary Tracey Ross fashion store in Los Angeles (8595 Sunset Boulevard, Los Angeles 90069; 310-854-1996), swears by Olga, the owner of the **Spa Kinara** (656 North Robertson Boulevard, Los Angeles 90069; 310-657-9188) who she says is the "best facialist in L.A." (and in case you're interested she says that Genia at the L.A. Four Seasons' hotel spa is the best manicurist and pedicurist). Meanwhile her friend, the British socialite Tamara Beckwith, goes to Tina at **Ole Henriksen** (8622 West Sunset Boulevard, Los Angeles 90069; 310-854-7700) for her twice-yearly facials and her lavender soaks (and for waxing to Michelle at Anastasia, 438 North Bedford Drive, Beverly Hills 90210; 310-273-3155, and to 1.a. vie l'orange, 638½ North Robertson Boulevard, Los Angeles 90069; 310-289-2501, for her pedicures).

Bliss Soho, 568 Broadway, New York 10012; www.bliss world.com (call 212-219-8970 for an appointment) and its many other branches around the country all offer a Triple Oxygen Facial Mask (not cheap at $160 for eighty-five minutes, but then needs must), which is a brilliant reviver of dingy skin.

Natura Bissé, which hails from Barcelona and makes gorgeous products, is a newish brand to the United States. Its facial (you get it for free if you spend $300 worth of products at the Natura Bissé spa at Bergdorf Goodman, 212-753-7300) leaves the skin looking truly radiant.

Eve Lom, 2 Spanish Place, Marylebone, London W1U 3HU; +44 20 7935 9988, is legendary, generally being agreed to offer the gold standard for facials—her fans book up months in advance. If you know you're coming to London it's well worth writing her into your schedule and in the meantime you can try her famous Cleansing Balm and her little muslin cloths.

There are a couple of other jewels if you're coming to England—**Anastasia Achilleos** is one of London's best-kept secrets. She has a gem of a salon in the basement of the San Domenico Hotel, 29–31 Draycott Place, London SW3 25H (call +44 7939 331 889 for an appointment). It's filled with all manner of delicious lotions and potions, with which she works many kinds of facial and massage magic, charging £150 ($300) for ninety minutes.

The Organic Pharmacy, 396 King's Road, London SW10 0LN (call +44 20 7351 2232 for an appointment), and Michaeljohn, 25 Albermarle Street, London W1S 4HU (for an appointment call +44 20 7629 6969), which has linked up with the Organic Pharmacy, both offer some of the same treatments, using the Organic Pharmacy's beautiful, mainly natural products. Ask for the Rose Crystal Lymphatic Facial. Too many late nights and too much alcohol leaves the lymph system stressed. The combination of rose crystals and acupressure massage to move the toxins around the lymphatic system revitalizes the skin. Also included in the treatment is deep cleansing, exfoliation, steaming, extraction, and four luxurious masks (Rose Hip, Seaweed, Honey and Jasmine, and Collagen) as well as massage of the hands, arms, feet, face, décolletage, and scalp, which incorporates a nourishing hair serum. The result is really glowing skin (and very messy hair—book a hair appointment for afterward). It takes ninety minutes and costs about $200.

Eyes

I am unable to endure much in the way of creams and lotions anywhere near my eyes, as they make them red and weepy. But there are a whole host of specialist creams that claim to do wonders for that sensitive area and undoubtedly some of them are effective for some women—just not for me. If your eyes are

Do-It-Yourself

If you can't get to the salons I've mentioned, here are some products that will help you to do a similar job at home. **The Organic Pharmacy's Collagen Boost Mask** ($110), although not as brilliant as the Rose Crystal Facial (nothing else is, in my view), is a good do-it-yourself rescue remedy. Try, too, the delicious-smelling **Rose Plus Face Cream**—though expensive at $210, it really seems to lighten and plump up the skin.

From **Bliss** (www.blissworld.com) there's the **Steep Clean Mask** ($54), a fifteen-minute do-it-yourself facial in a tube. It'll unclog the skin, remove dead cells (the chief culprit in making skin look dull), refine the pores and brighten the surface of the skin. Its **Instant Mattification Gel** ($36) is a sort of gel powder, which gives a beautiful finished look to the skin. But for really instant brightening, try the **Laboratoire Remède Double Oxygenating Booster** ($95). It pumps out fresh oxygen as well as alpha- and beta-hydroxy acids, which, say the boys and the girls in the white coats, is what brightens up the skin. You should notice a difference straightaway. It can be applied morning and evening and is particularly good if your skin is oily or prone to spots. If you can be bothered, there's also a **Laboratoire Remède Skin Exacting Mask** ($88), which exfoliates (removing all those dead cells that you don't want hanging about), refines and smoothes.

I'm also a fan of **Jurlique's Herbal Recovery Gel**, which really is a tonic for those days when your skin feels duller than the gray sky.

sensitive like mine, look for beauty lines that are hypoallergenic. What I do find works are the new generation of serums, which specially target the thinner, more sensitive skin around the eyes. Eye gels, too, are lighter and seem to irritate my eyes less. Two new recent products have proved lifesavers for me on the eye front—Natura Bissé's Diamond Extreme Eye (about $250), which I can use without my eyes becoming irritated or puffy and which really seems to help, and Crème de la Mer's Eye Balm ($180), which also works for me.

However, there are lots of things that can make your eyes look great.

First, get your brows professionally done. You can always tell a high-maintenance woman because her brows are always perfect. Eyebrows and pedicures have, for my money, to be among the cheapest of beauty treatments that really do make an impact. Getting your brows done at one of the many good salons around the country or in New York at somewhere like Alexis Vogel (www.makeupbyalexis.com) or Carmindy (www.carmindy.com) will give you a proper shape, which you can try and follow with your own tweezers afterwards.

In London, Linda Meredith (36 Beauchamp Place, London SW3 1NU; +44 20 7225 2755; www.lindameredith.com), eyebrow plucker to the stars, only costs just over $40 but, oh, the difference. These days you can walk into many department stores and get your brows done as soon as a technician is free. Londoners can go to Harvey Nichols's Beyond Beauty on the ground floor and get Blink's Indian threading service for $30. Fenwick of New Bond Street offers a similar service. At Selfridges, Groom will do eyebrows and lots more. (They offer high-speed treatments for those short of time where two therapists will work on a customer at once—one doing, say, eyebrows and a facial, the other doing a pedicure.)

If your eyebrows are beginning to thin out—oh, the woes of getting older—many salons nowadays offer tattooing (or to use the more official terminology—micropigmentation). This needs to be skillfully done if they're to look natural. In New York Denise DeGiulio (see page 106) is an expert—so expert that she's the one students turn to learn from. In London Debra Robson-Lawrence (144 Harley Street, London W1G 7LE; +44 845 230 2021; www.permanent-makeup.com) does wonderfully natural-looking tattoos.

Be warned: for the first two weeks they look a bit strong—more John Bolton than Greta Garbo—but they quickly soften to look more natural. Debra specializes in permanent makeup of all kinds and will also tattoo very gently around the lips, giving you an amazingly plump-looking mouth without the need of fillers (so no risk, then, of looking like a gasping goldfish).

A good tip from Bobbi Brown—it's better to use a soft brush and some eye shadow to define the brows rather than a pencil, which leaves a rather harsher line.

Tips for Eyes

White eyeliner inside the inner lid, if you can stand it, is brilliant for masking the pink of the inner eyelid. Estée Lauder, in particular, has a great Artist's Eye Pencil ($18.50).

Novalash (www.novalash.com) goes in for what it calls "eyelash enhancement"—that is, adding false eyelashes to your own to make them look lusher. Although very effective, they only last as long as your own eyelashes.

For puffy eyes, facial lymph drainage therapy is worth a try and most good facialists offer this during the normal course of a treatment. This therapy boosts circulation, and helps to eliminate toxins as well as make the face look firmer.

Necks and Chests

Nora Ephron, that wonderfully witty author of the screenplay for *When Harry Met Sally,* has, with her latest book, *I Feel Bad About My Neck,* given vent to one great cry of anguish about the sags, wrinkles and droops that come with the territory of being middle-aged. Quite obviously, it's her neck that bothers her most. (She's photographed on the cover wearing a black turtleneck sweater, a good ploy that the rest of us might copy, at least until global warming hits us.) "Dear Nora," I feel like telling her, "there are things that help" (though, to be truthful, the only cure for very saggy skin on the neck is plastic surgery, about which more on page 137).

As you get older, the two hardest areas to fix are the tops of the arms, and the décolletage and neck. Though we can cover them up for long chunks of the year, come summer vacation, heat waves, time on the beach or around the pool, all is revealed.

Upper arms (if you can face it—it doesn't quite seem worth it to me) can be dealt with by SmartLipo (a quick, lighter form of liposuction). But much can be done, you'll be happy to hear, to improve the décolletage. I had mine much improved at the Soma Centre, a charming spa and gym in the basement of the Royal Garden Hotel at 2–24 Kensington High Street, London W8 4PY (+44 7765 850 924), but lots of clinics now offer specialist techniques. Dr. Jules Nabet, a French cosmetic doctor, and aesthetician Joanne Evans have joined forces to offer a double-pronged attack on this vexed area. They use a combination of Botox and laser therapy. The two treatments together cost about $800, so not cheap, but they make a serious difference. They remove brown spots, plump up the skin and deal with creases. You need to plan ahead because, to begin with, there will be some reddening and darkening of the spots, and it takes two weeks for this to clear completely.

There is also now another weapon in the chest wars—RioBlush Carboxy Therapy. To put it at its simplest it involves injecting carbon dioxide beneath the skin with a fine needle—this causes blood vessels to dilate and forces extra oxygen to rush into the area bringing with it nutrients, encouraging collagen production and making the skin look firmer and fatter. It originated in Rio, is a huge success in the United States while in the U.K. only the Soma Centre so far offers it.

Other treatments for rejuvenating the neck and chest include Restylane Vital, which is very good for surface wrinkling, Botox (to deal with wrinkling caused by muscle action), and photo-rejuvenation techniques to tackle sun spots and red or brown blemishes on the surface of the skin. Dr. Nabet also recommends using a prescription-strength retinoid such as Retin-A (a cream) or Tazarotene (a gel), and utters the usual mantra: "Don't go out in the sun without a proper sunscreen."

Dr. Bryan Forley has been using Fraxel on the décolletage with very good results (5 East Eighty-second Street, New York 10028; 212-861-3757; www.drforley.com).

Most good aesthetic practices keep up to date with all the latest treatments—it's a mighty competitive business after all—but here are two good practices that I have personal experience of that you could check out in New York.

Dr. Howard Sobel, 960 Park Avenue, New York 10028; 212-288-0060, offers everything from Botox and Restylane injections to microdermabrasion, liposuction, glycolic peels, as well as lots of rather more esoteric treatments. On top of all that he also deals with more serious medical matters such as cancers, acne and the like.

Dr. Steven Victor, found at Victor Dermatology & Rejuvenation PC (30 East Seventy-sixth Street, New York 10021; 212-249-3050; www.stevenvictormdmedispa.com) is rumored to be the "derm" made famous by Plum Sykes's book *Bergdorf*

Blondes. He's certainly skillful, experienced, and attends to the beauty needs, whether the nonsurgical face-lift, Botox, Restylane, laser work, SmartLipo, or peels, of all manner of chic New York socialites.

Then there are neck creams. Some women swear by them, and I'm of the view that all nourishment helps the skin, but until I tried Nature Bissé's Inhibit-Tensolift (which really seems to work and does not seem too oily or creamy), I found them too tricky to use. It was just one step too far for me and the cream seemed to get onto my clothes or bed linen. Committed beauty junkies, who can find the time to deal with every niche problem, no doubt have other creams that work for them. Me, I like a simpler routine, and I'm afraid that if I run out of Nature Bissé's Tensolift, my neck is rather left to look after itself as best it can.

MAKEUP

The chief thing to remember is that *you can always wash it off.* Some women seem to treat makeup as if it were a dangerous innovation that might leave them permanently impaired. Most skins look better, in my view, with some makeup. As we get older our coloring tends to fade and makeup helps to lift the face. Those with sallow complexions that need a little lifting and added coloring benefit particularly. Good foundations (there are masses but my two current favorites are Giorgio Armani's Designer Shaping Cream Foundation SPF 20 and Estée Lauder's Resilience Lift Extreme) even out the skin tone, hide light blemishes and give the skin a certain luminous quality.

The older you get, though, the less good you look with powder—it settles in the creases—so these days I'm very fond of Serge Lutens Teint Si Fin, a compressed all-in-one makeup in eight different shades that is dabbed on with a sponge and gives a smooth, flawless, natural finish. It's all part of his very edited, very small line of makeup called Nécessaires de Beauté, designed to give that Holy Grail of the makeup world: the no-makeup look (see page 117). It's devilishly hard to track down but you can buy it online at www.salons-shiseido.com. Mind you the Shiseido shop in the Palais Royale in Paris is such a gem that it is worth visiting it if only to sniff Serge Lutens's perfumes and to try the makeup for yourself. It has to be said that they are very expensive indeed, which is why I am now turning more frequently to the Bare Escentuals Bare Minerals line—its Bare Minerals Foundation is perfect for giving the no-makeup look and is a fraction of the price. Valentine Alexander describes it as "the Maserati of mineral makeup—easy, quick and modern." Go to www.bareescentuals.com to find out more.

Every face is different and skin tones vary enormously, so most of us need to experiment to find out what suits us. All the big makeup brands are a wonderful source of information, though only for their own products. You can get your makeup done at their counters for free, which is a wonderful service and shows you just how makeup should be applied. Turn up at a big store—Bloomingdale's, Saks, Nordstrom, Neiman's, or one near where you live—take your place in the line, if there is one, and you can learn a lot. Otherwise there is nothing for it but either a bit of personal experimenting or a lesson from a makeup artist.

Possibly the most important thing to get right is foundation. If the color is wrong, it spoils the whole look. Textures vary considerably, too, and I'm afraid that only trial and error can help you find the right foundation for you.

Primers

Primers are relative newcomers on the beauty scene. The point of them is that they help prepare the skin, refining the pores and smoothing the skin, providing a better surface for the foundation so that it "takes" more easily. I have friends who swear by primers from Trish McEvoy and Laura Mercier. I'm using one by Trish McEvoy, and it does make a difference.

Radiance

Radiance, you might think, has been around for a long time. Natural radiance has, yes, but when it comes to cosmetics, new technical discoveries—most particularly light-reflecting particles—have helped the beauty companies develop products that are specifically targeted at giving you a more radiant skin. I'm keen on them—and who wouldn't be?

There are radiance-boosting moisturizers to apply under makeup, like Estée Lauder's Daywear Plus Sheer Tint Release Formula, which definitely gives the skin a more luminous look, as well as plenty of others. Just look for products that have magic words on the packages, like "light reflecting," "luminizers" or "brightening."

Here are three products that I believe really help: Guerlain's Midnight Star, Liz Earle's Brightening Treatment, and B. Kamins Diatomamus Earth Masque.

> ☞ *A great tip for adding radiance, which comes from an eminent Hollywood makeup artist: put a little of your foundation into the palm of your hand, add a tiny (and she means tiny) drop of glycerine, and mix well before applying. It will give a gorgeous glow to the skin without making it greasy.*

For the No-Makeup Look

Tinted moisturizers are all some skins need. For instance, Estée Lauder's Daywear Plus Multi-Protection Antioxidant Moisturizer Sheer Tint (with an SPF of 15) is a good one. Many other beauty companies produce very light formulations for those who don't need much cover. Origins Nude and Improved Bare Face Makeup (with an SPF of 15) is good because it offers just a little more cover-up than most, and comes in five shades (www.origins.com).

Chantecaille's Real Skin (which has an SPF of 30) and Future Skin manage to be incredibly light while evening out skin texture and covering up blemishes. And then of course there's the already mentioned Bare Escentuals Bare Mineral Foundation, while Laura Mercier's very new range requires nothing but a couple of licks of powdered mineral foundation—quick, easy, and perfect.

The chief tactic in the no-makeup look is to apply foundation (or perhaps even just a good concealer) only where you have blemishes, broken veins or brown spots, and leave unblemished skin clear of makeup altogether. Blend the foundation or concealer carefully so that it's impossible to tell where the skin starts and the foundation ends. I think foundations that are a mix of cream and powder together—there are now many—look lighter than those that need powder to fix them. If you must use powder, choose a transparent one and brush it on lightly. Finish with a light lip gloss.

Need a Bit of Cover-up?

Avoid (unless you have deep port-wine birthmarks) all those medical cover-up creams—they're much too heavy. These days there are lighter, cleverer ways to conceal.

There's a whole new generation of concealers that make some of the old favorites look heavy and masklike in comparison. Guerlain's Issima Precious Light Smoothing Illuminator has high-tech pigments and pearly particles that make it a pretty magic product. It masks blemishes and lines as well as offering a good base for those with skin problems.

Otherwise Jane Iredale (www.janeiredale.com) is the magic name to remember if you need to cover up anything from acne scars to red veins. A good moisturizer to start with is her Absence ($35.50), which has an SPF of 15 and built-in oil control. Its light-reflecting properties seem to diminish as well as fill in the scars. If there are any outstanding blotches or scars, stipple on Jane Iredale's Circle/Delete ($29). Finish off with Iredale's Amazing Base ($24) in a shade to suit your skin tone. Most spas and natural cosmetics stores sell her products.

Beauty on the Cheap

Great makeup brands to look for if you want to save the pennies are Bourjois (which is made by Chanel—say no more) and L'Oreal (which makeup guru Valentine Alexander says is very similar to Lancôme). L'Oreal is stocked in every supermarket and drug store, and you can find Bourjois at Sephora and Ulta. Nivea, Olay, and Roc are the best inexpensive, low-priced, skin-care lines while Liz Earle is wonderful value.

Makeup Specialists

Here are a few that I know to be good from personal experience:

IN THE UNITED STATES
Alexis Vogel (www.makeupbyalexis.com, to book call 818-519-7790) is credited with doing the makeup for many a red

carpet habitué (such as Pamela Anderson and Sharon Stone) but you, too, can get to share her secrets by booking in (via the Web site or by telephone) and have a makeup devised specially for you. Cheap, she ain't. She offers two packages—one is makeup plus lesson and hair styling for $2,500 and the other is makeup and lesson plus hair color, new cut, and style for $3,000. But you could get a face chart, digital photographs and Polaroid pictures to take home and remind you what to do.

Carmindy is best known for working with Isabella Rossellini and Cindy Crawford, but she's also done many a beauty shoot with most major magazines. A one-and-a-half-hour consultation would include brow grooming and learning which makeup is right for you and how to apply it. She will also go through your makeup bag and tell you what to keep and what to throw. If you can't afford the fee ($1,000), her Web site (www.carmindy.com) is wonderfully informative and packed with helpful hints.

Denise DeGiulio owns and runs Enhanced Image at 130 West Fifty-seventh Street, Suite 10F, New York 10019 (212-957-0777), and besides being the best-regarded expert for micropigmentation (finely tattooing eyebrows, lips, etc.) she will give you a makeup plan devised especially for you.

Kimara Ahnert—credited with helping many a mover and shaker with their glossy looks (Catherine Zeta-Jones, Marla Maples, and Brooke Shields to name but three)—has her makeup studio (1113 Madison Avenue, New York 10028; 212-452-4252) in a sumptuously furnished townhouse, all plush mirrors, antique sofas, and Aubusson rugs. She'll give you a complete skin-care regime, tweak the eyebrows, wax the legs, but she'll also devise a makeup scheme just for you. She also works with lots of plastic surgeons and dermatologists for those who want or need more serious work done. She'll give you a makeup lesson for $250, but you could have one of her highly trained assistants for $185.

IN THE U.K.

Valentine Alexander is, in my view, worth every penny of the some $500 she charges. She sees the face as a canvas and treats it in rather the same way Renaissance portrait painters did. Because she isn't tied to a particular beauty house, she uses what she considers the best products for the purpose. Since some of these are very expensive, she can help you avoid buying the wrong one. She comes to London a few times a month and offers advice at her studio in Knightsbridge, and in Paris. Call her respectively at +44 7956 846 909 and at +33 6 99 63 34 10 to book an appointment.

Stephen Glass at Face Facts is very nice indeed and gentle, and he does makeup brilliantly. Like Valentine, he cruises all the beauty houses for what he considers to be the best products. Contact him on +44 7753 616 617 or e-mail him on contact@stephenglass.co.uk.

Maggie Hunt has addressed the makeup problems of such luminaries as Shakira Caine, Helen Mirren, Baroness Thatcher, Vanessa Redgrave, and Maggie Smith, and if she's good enough for them I'm sure she's great for the rest of us. "It's from forty-five and upwards," she says, "that my clients need most help. They're usually using too heavy an eyeliner, lots of mascara and too heavy a foundation while missing out on the blusher." Her best product for lips? Lipfinity by Max Factor. Her studio is in Hampstead, where a two-hour makeup lesson costs around $500. Call +44 20 7435 5049 for an appointment (also at www.maggiehunt.com).

Neisha Hibbert will devise makeup regimes for clients in her own South Kensington house (+44 7768 078 766 for an appointment) for $150, but if you are in London, she will also come to you for $300.

Daniel Sandler, who's been doing faces for photographic shoots for many a long year, will also come to you (or send one of his own personally trained makeup artists) to hold a master class in how to apply makeup. A more glamorous kind of Tupperware party, if you like. You need a minimum of five friends and he charges less than $200 per person, which includes a glass of champagne. He not only goes through the makeup you already own (be prepared for some stringent comments) but passes on all those little tips that only insiders usually acquire. He guides you on how to find the right color of concealer (most of us choose too pale a color—it should match our foundation), how to sculpt cheekbones, and lots, lots more. Call +44 1923 845 370 or check www.danielsandler.com.

Sarah Chapman is a makeup artist much favored by *The Times* fashion desk (+44 7050 097 796).

John Gustafson at Fenwick of New Bond Street (+44 20 7629 9161) has a waiting list longer than my arm (about three years to be precise), but you could plan ahead and book way in advance.

TEETH

Good teeth do more to take the years off than almost anything else—and they can also be life-changing, affecting both career and romantic prospects. There are now clinics all over the land that will whiten your teeth, straighten them, cap them and—if you can afford the gold standard—give you light, pearly-perfect veneers. While teeth whitening with a laser costs about $800 all in, crowns cost $750 upward per tooth and pearly veneers about $600 per tooth. So this kind of dentistry is not cheap but if your teeth are bad, my goodness, the difference it makes.

The first time I had mine whitened it was at the surgery of the divine Marc Lowenberg and Gregg Lituchy (Lowenberg & Lituchy, 230 Central Park South, New York 10019;

212-586-2890; www.lowenbergandlituchy.com), the providers of perfect pearlies to New York's uptown set, as well as untold luminaries of stage and screen. Since I was merely in town for a few days whitening was all that was possible (the Rolls-Royce treatment, state-of-the-art perfection is opalescent porcelain-fine veneers, which take more time). The great advantage of veneers is that once they're in, that's the color they stay for the duration, anything from ten to twenty years. Nicotine, coffee, and red wine pass them smoothly by. For those who have crooked or chipped teeth, gaps or sharp points, the porcelain veneers deal with the lot. I tried the relatively new and fast laser-whitening procedure that took some two hours and was brilliantly successful—I emerged with much whiter teeth. Since then, as I'm a tea and coffee addict and do like the odd glass of red wine, they have become slowly dingier with time.

After they'd lost their gorgeous whiteness I thought they needed redoing so I went to Dr. Joe Oliver at the Welbeck Clinic (20 Welbeck St., London W1G 8ED; +44 870 241 6903; www.thewelbeckclinic.co.uk). Since then things have speeded up. Dr. Oliver's Power Whitening treatment took one and a half hours from start to finish and it really worked, though the result may vary from person to person.

There is a fast system for veneers, called CEREC, which is ready after only one visit to the dentist. Cerec veneers are supposedly stronger than the usual porcelain ones and last as long as thirty years. Most veneers take a minimum of two weeks to make, which is usually enough for most of us, but it's nice to know that if you have a serious emergency (a film premiere? a wedding? a vital job interview?), they can be done in a day. You can see the dentist one day, pick the veneers up the next.

Hair

Nothing—not even a pair of Manolo Blahniks or a blissful shearling coat—does more for the morale than a spanking new haircut that really works. (We will pass lightly over those occasions, an inevitable part of the female rite of passage, when you rush scarlet-faced straight from the hairdresser to the sink at home.) A great cut can transform the plain into the glamorous, the scruffy into the glossy, and the merely pretty into a beauty. Think Chelsea Clinton, once an ugly duckling, these days a glossy beauty, and her revamped hair is a large part of the newly acquired glamour. Some women find their style early on and stick with it—look no further than Anna Wintour. Others reinvent themselves eternally.

The secret of the right cut, though, is elusive—not helpful, I'm afraid, but true—for it depends more upon art, a sensitive eye and intuitive scissors than just technique. Tastes need to mesh so that the crimper's idea of chic or glamour matches yours. There are a few legendary cutters around—John Barrett in New York (754 Fifth Avenue, New York 10019; 212-872-2700), for whom jet setters run up phenomenal quantities of hair-miles, and Christophe Robin in Paris (9 rue Guénégaud, Paris 75006; +33 1 42 60 99 15), for whom several Londoners regularly cross the Channel. John Sahag of New York (425 Madison Avenue, New York 10017; 212-750-7772) also has a cult following and gave my best-dressed New York friend a haircut to die for, although he failed to do the same for me. Some years ago Richard at the 4th Floor (4 Northington Street, London WC1N 2JG; +44 20 7405 6011) gave me the cut that most transformed my look, creating a shortish helmet of hair that swirled and shone, and made something of a stir back in the office. (I try to forget the other time a haircut of mine caused a kerfuffle at conference time, when a well-known crimper gave me a disastrous perm.)

Readers might like to know that many a London socialite turns, as do I, to Hari at Hari's, 305 Brompton Road, London SW3 2DY (+44 20 7581 5211) for salvation when their tresses need tending. Rebecca (who does my color) is a genius and Hari effortlessly somehow turns my not-very-promising locks into something passably chic. He now has a hair spa, which translates into a whole lot of TLC for the hair. Turn up and they'll tell you which of their many treatments will restore it if it is stressed, tired, overworked or simply freaked out by environmental damage. I've also recently had a great cut from Paul Edmonds who gave me a completely sassier, new chic cut. He's at 217 Brompton Road, London SW3; +44 20 7589 5958.

The golden rule about hair has to be that if you see somebody with a haircut you admire, ask who did it. After I first got that wonderful short helmet (I was *much* younger then), I was endlessly stopped and asked—most notably while boarding a plane in Hong Kong—and was always flattered. Then go for it. Don't hang on to straight long tresses because once, long ago, somebody admired them. Nothing is more aging or dates you more. Sometimes the transformation is effected in one fell swoop. Sometimes it takes a few visits to the hairdresser before enough trust has built up to let the cutter have his or her wicked way. Watch carefully what he does for others—if you like it, the chances are he'll suit you, too.

As for color, go for that too, if you need it. The fashion at the moment is for thick chunky streaks (known as "slicing" in the trade) rather than ultrafine ones (Jennifer Aniston, Cameron Diaz). A great cut, a new color, with some of the splendid new products that help preserve the shine, can update a look more quickly than a Marc Jacobs jacket.

But don't always stick to conventional thinking about hair. Take the example of Evelyn Lauder, wife of Leonard Lauder and a formidable person in her own right. When I interviewed her a couple of years ago, she told me that she had recently decided to "reinvent myself. I'd been wearing my hair short for years and one day when I had a brilliant cut at Coppola in Milan [the branch near the main Armani store, in case you're interested], I just decided it was so good that I didn't want to cut it short again." So she gently grew it out and it gave her a new softer, very pretty look—overturning the convention that as you get older you should cut your hair shorter. "The key," says Mrs. Lauder, "is keeping your hair in good condition so that it shines. I do color my hair but use no peroxide." In New York, Kao at AKS (694 Madison Avenue, New York 10021; to book an appointment call 212-888-0707), she told me, kept it looking good.

As you grow older, getting the color attended to can take years off your appearance. As the hair changes color so, too, does the skin—you need a really gifted colorist to get it right. A few women look wonderful with their hair a particularly chic shade of steel gray, but most of us turn a speckled gray and white, and quite often the gray is yellowish—not a pretty look! So don't just drift along—get it attended to. If you spend money on nothing else, spend it on your hair. Don't hold back out of timidity. If you don't try something new, you'll never know whether it will work or not and at the end of the day you can always grow it out.

☞ SERIOUS HELP *Almost every hairdresser offers good masks and conditioning treatments. I believe that if you can afford it, it's worth having them—they're rather like facials in that they nourish and restore. These, however, are almost the easiest treatments to do yourself at home, which is so much cheaper. Kérastase is about the best home-hairdressing line around but Shu Uemura's got a new range out (Art of Hair) which has three lines for colored, damaged or dry hair and it is fantastic. For real hair loss (alopecia), you need medical help.*

Hands

Hands are a big giveaway on the age front, although that might not worry you. After all, most of us aren't trying to con the world into believing we're younger than we are; we just want to look the best we can—but hands that aren't looked after can actually look a whole lot *older* than we are, which I think it's perfectly permissible to dislike. If you had nothing else to do and your night-life is unexciting, you could wear Bliss Glamour Gloves every night—they come ready infused with a nourishing grapeseed and ceramide gel to moisturize and nourish, check out www.blissworld.com. You could also exfoliate your hands, use peels and scrubs on them, and pamper them with enriching creams. Most of us have rather more interesting (or pressing) things to do so it's worth simplifying things a bit.

First, get a hand cream (we all need one, don't we?) that has a high SPF so that your hands are protected from sun damage as much as possible. It's the sun that mostly causes the aging brown spots. Given that prevention is easier than cure, if you're young and don't yet have age spots, you should start using hand creams with in-built SPFs *before* they appear. We all think it's only other people who get these things—but believe me, it's not true.

If you already have brown spots, it's probably worth investing in a few serious treatments; getting rid of them makes a big difference. Go to a good aesthetic treatment centre (they are now all over the country) and get them zapped. It's dead easy. Microdermabrasion and IPL treatments will really improve the look of your hands and will boost their collagen, too. You can also have a chemical peel to even out the skin tone and make the skin softer, while Thermage will tighten the skin. Afterwards, just take care to nourish your hands regularly, look after your nails with a good hand and nail cream, and keep the UV rays at bay. There are newer treatments around now that aim to plump up the skin—Restylane, Fraxel, and fat injections can all be used to make the hands seem less scrawny and therefore younger.

Hand creams that I like: Clarins's Hand and Nail Treatment Cream; Lancôme's Caresse Mains; and Liz Earle's Hand Repair, which has a good texture and smells pleasantly herbal. Crème de la Mer now has a hand cream and I love it, too, but there are lots and lots that all work well. If you're hard-up don't spend too much on hand creams—choose one with an SPF of 15 or more and that makes your skin feel good.

Nails

I was much comforted to learn that the late Liz Tilberis, an editor at U.K. *Vogue* and latterly editor of *Harper's Bazaar,* never had a manicure until she reached her fifties. Americans, we know, have always been way ahead of the Brits on the grooming front and it obviously helps that on every corner, certainly in New York and probably in most big cities, there are wonderful salons that will give blow-dries, manis, and pedis without an appointment at prices that most working girls can afford. I always envy great nails, for I've never successfully cracked the problem of nails that split and although I find that nail polish makes them look wonderful while it's on, my nails are much brittler and drier a few weeks later. I find the Barielle group of products for nails the best (800-790-8884 and at www.barielle.com).

I once consulted a serious nutritionist (Lorraine Perretta, a quick-talking New Yorker who now mostly works in Britain) about healthy eating and when I took the vast quantity of nutritional supplements that she prescribed, my nails were noticeably better. The downside was that they all took a lot of swallowing each day (there was zinc, calcium, potassium, plus an array of vitamins) and I rather feebly gave up. But if you can keep it up, it will make a difference and, as Lorraine Perretta puts it, "if it makes that much difference to your nails just think what it's doing to everything else—your bones, your hair, your skin, your muscles."

French manicures are now considered tacky, but I still think it useful to run Sally Hansen's Nail White Pencil (about $2) under your nails to give a good clean look at the tip. Track down a good manicurist and get your nails regularly looked after. It isn't very expensive, and it's well worth it.

Legs

The things that make a difference are:

1. **Genes**, about which you can do nothing.

2. **Exercise**, about which you can do a lot; some is essential to keep legs well toned.

3. **Eating well**, lots of fresh fruit and vegetables, and drinking lots of water. This is not always compatible with real life, but there you go, that's this beauty lark for you.

4. **Body brushing**, yes, really. I've never had the patience to do it but those who daily brush their legs very lightly (just enough to move the lymph along), brushing upwards from the feet toward the heart, report marked improvements. This is especially essential for those with the dimpled skin that we call cellulite.

5. **Creams.** I've never had the time, patience, or willpower to apply daily creams that are specially targeted at improving skin texture or dealing with cellulite. However, more dedicated seekers after perfection than I report that if you keep at it stolidly (and I really mean stolidly: it takes something like six months), you will see some improvement.

6. **Massage**, particularly for those with cellulite, as it helps move the toxins along.

7. **Mesotherapy**. Some people believe in it although when I tried it, it did nothing for my most troublesome area (my stomach), and it also requires lots of treatments before you see any real improvement. Worth a go, but I'm a bit dubious myself.

8. **Grooming**. Most obviously of all, keep your legs well waxed and, in summer, brown, using bronzers or home-tanning sprays or creams. All the best-groomed young women I know tell me that many a beauty swears by Rodial's Brazilian Tan lotion—find it at Space NK and Bliss.

FEET

These days most of us are much more alert to the joys of a proper pedicure than ever before. Partly this is due to the rise and rise of vertiginously expensive shoes (Jimmy Choo, Manolo Blahnik, Prada, Louis Vuitton, and all the other usual suspects), which has meant that it seemed like sartorial sacrilege to put ugly, gnarled old toes into such delicious concoctions. There are now good nail salons in almost every shopping center and pedicures aren't rocket science, so most of them probably do a good job.

If you have serious foot problems (bunions, ingrown toenails, corns, and the like) you need a podiatrist and the United States, you will not be surprised to learn, is not short of highly qualified experts. Dr. Oliver Zong (80 Maiden Lane, Suite 703, New York 10038; 212-385-2400) and Dr. Suzanne Levine, who works out of the Institute Beauté (885 Park Avenue, New York 10075; 212-535-0229), are two of the best-known.

Although I'm not good at this as I'm always in too much of a hurry, I'd add to that—do try to rub the hard skin off your feet regularly. On their Web site, Jo Fairley and Sarah Stacey

rave about the Alida Foot File (about $20 from www.victoria
health.com, which ships to the United States), saying it is the
best foot file they've ever come across. It's ergonomically designed and easy to use.

Bliss SoHo, 568 Broadway, New York 10012; 212-219-
8970, has lots of special foot treats, including its Rosy Toes
(sixty minutes for $70), which involves resting your feet on
warm stones and soaking them in rose-petal-strewn water. If
you have calluses, there's the "Hot Milk and Almond Pedicure"
(sixty minutes for $65), which offers "intensive dry-buffing
with a fierce callus fighter."

SPArties (877-772-7843 and at www.sparties.com). If
you're the girly sort, you can throw a pampering party where
you all experiment with foot soaks, exfoliators, and different

---

A pedicure is a much less serious matter but nevertheless few things deliver so much satisfaction for
so little outlay. For something like $50 you can
emerge from most salons with some immaculately
primped toes. But it's even cheaper—and not
difficult—to do it yourself. Iris Chapple, one of
London's most sought-after pedicurists, gave me
the run-down on how to do it at home. Here it is:

"Brush your skin when it's dry. Never use nail
hardeners. They're the worst because they dry the
nails out. Keep some almond oil by the bed and put
a drop on each nail (hands and feet) every night.
Cut nails straight across. Never use corn plasters—
always go to a podiatrist to have corns treated. Many
of the inexpensive products are just as good as the
expensive ones. Maybelline polish, for instance, at
about [$3] a bottle, is just as good as more expen-
sive makes, and it has a brilliant high shine."

polishes. SPArties offers a menu of different pampering treats (including facials and massages), and you can get a therapist for $100 for an hour, or for $300 a guest, you could get your home turned into a spa—complete with robes and relaxing ambience—which sounds like fun.

Pedicures Around the World

Bastien Gonzalez is probably the world's most famous specialist, the Bastien experience being unlike any other. He did my feet when he still had a treatment room at Claridge's in London (55 Brook Street, London W1K 4HX) and it is much, much more than a pedicure. In fact, he doesn't even paint the nails. He buffs and smoothes and shines the feet so that they don't even *need* to be painted. He's a bit peripatetic so you need to track him down to make an appointment in advance. In London these days he works out of the Cadogan Hotel, 75 Sloane Street, London SW1X 9SG; +44 0 20 7235 7141. Check his Web site at www.bastien gonzalez.com and e-mail for an appointment.

Mr. So at the Mandarin Hotel, 5 Connaught Road, in Central Hong Kong (+852 2522 0111; www .mandarinoriental.com), is another cult name. Those who have his pedicure swear that their feet become a whole size smaller and many a client books in their feet when they book a hotel room.

At the Paris Four Seasons, 31 avenue George V, Paris 75008 (www.fourseasons.com), they do the most blissful French finish, and while at the **Ritz-Carlton** in Key Biscayne, 455 Grand Bay Drive, Key Biscayne, FL 33149; 305-365-4158 (www .ritzcarlton.com), there are armchairs that vibrate with speed and heat settings, and two therapists give you a simultaneous manicure and pedicure.

TOP BEAUTY TIPS

1. Keep out of the sun. Use a sunblock like DDF's almost chemical-free Organic Sunblock (www.ddfskincare.com) and, when possible, wear a hat as well.

2. Use a lip balm. The best are Kiehl's and Smith's Rosebud Salve (available at www.sephora.com) and Rose Petal Salve from the Rose & Co Apothecary (84 Main Street, Haworth, West Yorkshire BD22 8DP; +44 1535 646 830; www.roseapothecary.co.uk).

3. Best red lipsticks: Chanel's Rouge Noir and Yves Saint Laurent's Rouge Pur Lipstick No. 19.

4. Use a lip pencil to deal with lines around the lips that cause lipsticks to bleed (Mac's Spice is a wonderfully accommodating shade), but never use one darker than your lipstick. A makeup artist taught me to outline my lips *outside* the lipline with a concealer (Chanel's Correcteur Éclat or Yves Saint Laurent's classic Touche Éclat) to make your lips look fuller.

5. Take care of your skin when traveling. Elizabeth Arden's Eight Hour Cream has been around since the 1930s, and many a beauty still swears by it. I also love Prescriptives Flight Cream. Calvin Klein is apparently a great fan and buys it by the boxful.

6. Use an eyelash curler. The best is from Shu Uemura and is curved like eyelids.

7. Need to mask a spot or small flaw? Bobbi Brown's Creamy Concealer comes in lots of shades so you can match your skin color exactly. Cheaper still is Rimmel's Hide the Blemish.

8. If you need a real pick-me-up for the skin before, say, a wedding, a seriously big date, an appearance on the catwalk or the red carpet (well, you never know), CACI Chroma-Oxy is rumored to be the treatment that Renée Zellweger

had before the Globes. It offers first a microdermabrasion followed by an oxygen facial. It takes ninety minutes, costs $150, and leaves the skin looking fresh and glowing. There's no downtime at all. The flagship salon is the C2 Clinic in Hampstead, 11 Heath Street, London NW3 6TP; +44 20 7435 1554.

9. Chanel's Cils Magique Waterproof Mascara famously survived a birthing pool—it really does stay on through most watery occasions.

10. Sleep, sleep, and more sleep.

> *If you ever catch sight of yourself in a mirror*
> *looking a bit slouched you'll never do it again.*
> *Stand and sit up straight—it takes years off.*
> —Evelyn Lauder

Vitamin Injections

I first heard about vitamin cocktails from the lovely Janan Harb, ex-wife of the late King Fahd of Saudia Arabia and a famous beauty. She took one look at me and hauled me off to the Pasha Clinic, a small clinic just off London's Regent Street (37 Maddox Street, London W1S 2PP; +44 20 7226 3662) where she swears by the treatments. Janan is so keen on vitamin injections that she'd have them every day if she could. She first discovered them when she had some facial burns after a fire at her home and the vitamin injections healed the burns so well that she was left without a single scar. The treatments consist of a tiny little needle injecting micro amounts of nutrients into the skin all over the face. It is mildly uncomfortable but it doesn't take long—about fifteen minutes, at a guess. According to Dr. Menevse Kargin, a wonderful Turkish doctor turned aesthetician who runs the Pasha Clinic, the cocktail she uses has a broad range of essential micronutrients (amino acids, vitamins, mineral salts, and nucleotides) that are needed for the many complex cellular biochemical processes that are the basis of normal cellular activity.

I can only tell you that after my series of seven treatments I ran into somebody whom I've known for years who asked me what on earth I'd done as I looked so good. And a makeup artist who was doing my face for a professional photograph kept commenting on how well plumped up my skin was.

THE NONSURGICAL FACE-LIFT

These days there are many techniques to help in the antiaging war without resorting to the knife. The face ages largely because we lose plumpness from under the skin, which causes the skin to sag, rather like air going out of a balloon. It follows that if you can reflate the balloon (i.e., the skin), it will look plumper and younger, and the lines will fill out.

There are now many different fillers—Restylane, Botox, and Sculptra to name but three—which are used to fill out the sagging skin. The other technique in the age war is, of course, the face-lift, which works in the opposite way by cutting away the excess sagging skin and tightening it up.

When I heard that Dr. Steven Victor (Steven Victor Medispa, 30 East Seventy-sixth Street, New York 10021; 212-249-3050), dubbed Dr. Lookgood by his patients and allegedly the model for the favorite dermatologist of the "Bergdorf Blondes" (in Plum Sykes's book), was bringing overseas his techniques for what he calls his "nonsurgical face-lift," I was there in a flash, volunteering to be a guinea pig.

This is how it works: first, the patient is given a series of injections rather like those at the dentist. They don't hurt—

much—but they do render your mouth area numb. Then he sets to work with his fillers.

This is what he did for me in his medi-spa: Botox in the forehead, between the eyes, around the nose and eyes, as well as around the eyebrow to lift the brows and the upper eyelids. I was given injections of Sculptra in the dermis, the fat and muscle layers of the cheekbones, to plump up the area and so "lift the face." (Knowing which layers to inject into is, it seems, a vital part of the procedure's success.) This was followed by deeper injections of Sculptra into the fat layer and superficial muscle layer of the nasolabial lines (the so-called laugh lines), as well as superficial injections of Restylane into the dermis. The lips were plumped up a little with silicone to help fill in a down-turning of the mouth.

You go home looking worse than when you came in, with red marks, a numb mouth, a bit of bruising. But it all subsides in a couple of days and after a week you really begin to notice the difference. My face looked a lot fresher and younger. I had higher cheekbones. The lines, particularly running from nose to mouth, were much reduced and he managed to inject the Botox so that my eyelids didn't droop (my big fear about Botox). Lines on my forehead had disappeared so I could wear my hair off my face again (my forehead had been very lined for some time). I think it truly made a difference and several friends have remarked on how well I look.

The cost: about $5,400.

How long does it last? Well, it varies. The silicone in the lips will last ten years, the Sculptra about two years, the Botox from three to six months and the Restylane from six to twelve months. So to keep looking this way isn't cheap.

Over on the West Coast, home of surgically-enhanced beauties, eminent plastic surgeons have their practices on almost every block. Insider information is always best. All of them will offer the sort of procedures that Dr. Steven Victor did so successfully on me but I cannot emphasize enough what I have said before—the techniques are there for everybody who has mastered them but above and beyond technique you need a surgeon with sensitivity and a fine aesthetic sense. Ask around. Two of the best are said to be Dr. Brian Novack (reputed to be the knife behind the smooth skin, wide-open eyes, and firm necks of many a red-carpet habitué; 414 North Camden Drive, Suite 1010, Beverly Hills 90210; 310-888-8818) and Dr. Raj Kanodia of 414 North Camden Drive, Suite 801, Beverly Hills 90210; 310-276-3106.

Dr. Olivier de Frahan is another artist when it comes to fillers (Botox, Restylane, and the full face-lift) and the person that many a French film star and model whose future work depends on looking good turns to for all serious beauty advice. He works in London and Paris—call respectively +44 20 7730 7928 and +33 6 09 55 77 77 for an appointment.

Warning: As New York plastic surgeon and dermatologist Dr. Bryan Forley put it to me, simply because techniques are there doesn't mean it is always wise to avail oneself of them. My experience tells me that before submitting yourself to any of these procedures, you should investigate very carefully the work of the aesthetician. Do not just turn up at any salon and ask for work to be done. Avoid offers of lunchtime treatments. Check very carefully on the previous work of the aesthetician. Botox in the wrong place, too much Restylane, or too much Sculptra can result in the trout mouths, bizarrely high cheeks and startled looks or drooping eyes that we're all, sadly, becoming more accustomed to seeing. The techniques are easy to master but the aesthetics of judging how much and where to put them require a fine and sensitive eye. In the right hands, they can make a huge difference for the better. In the wrong hands, they can wreak disaster.

PLASTIC SURGERY:
SHOULD YOU OR SHOULDN'T YOU?

I've never understood why some people get so het up when the matter of plastic surgery is up for discussion. It's almost as if it were a matter of deep moral import, with the implication that there is something inherently morally superior about allowing the wrinkles to wrinkle and the frowns to furrow and the droopy bits to get droopier. Not unlike some intellectuals who think it's a sign of a superior brain to dress in drab clothes.

Plastic surgery seems to me to be fundamentally a physical issue and, providing you're not proposing to pay for it by swiping the bread from your children's mouths, I cannot see that it is a moral issue at all. What good plastic surgery does is to cut away sagging bits of skin. It removes bags from under the eyes, droopiness from the top eyelids (not a good look, bloodhound eyelids), sagginess from the chin, and generally tightens up the skin. That's it. Now where's the problem with all of that? Of course, it is major surgery and does involve a general anesthesia so that needs to be taken into serious account. And if it's badly done, it's a hideously expensive mistake, but these days it seems to me that surgeons are getting better and better at it—heaven knows they're getting more practice. The general notion that it would be better to put up with age spots, red veins, droops, and sags when there is something that can be done about them seems to me just plain daft.

Nobody who looks at the before and after pictures of such success stories as Julie Christie, Jane Fonda, or Sharon Osbourne could surely still take the view that in their shoes they wouldn't have done the same. All three—and there are thousands of others like them—look a million times better and happier now that the damage the years can do has been held back a little longer. And for all three it's opened up professional opportunities that might not otherwise have come their way.

The usual charge by those who get all snooty at the very idea is that it speaks of vanity. Well, first, I see nothing wrong with vanity. Vanity makes us try harder; vanity makes us strive in many areas of our lives; vanity makes us look better, which adds considerably to the gaiety of the nation. But there is more than vanity at stake. Quite often these days it is often a matter of job survival. As we all live longer and longer (hurrah!) we want to go on living full and busy lives, and if we want to do that, it is no use denying that looks count. Whether you're behind the counter in a shop, working in a lawyer's office, trying to hold your own in the world of fashion, or running a small business, how you are seen by the outside world will affect your prospects.

These days there is a bewildering array of often very technical options for us to choose from, ranging from the surgeon's knife to lasers, light pulses, fillers, acid peels—the list is endless. Many things can now be treated: from sun-damaged skin to brown spots, red veins, dubious moles, excess hair, and many other afflictions. And if treatments exist that will deal with the things that indubitably make women feel less confident about themselves, I cannot for the life of me believe that it is anything other than a good idea to have them attended to.

Some of you may be frightened of the surgeon's knife—and not without reason. Mistakes are sometimes made (it must be almost impossible to estimate the damage that Mrs. Wildenstein alone must have done to the world of cosmetic surgery) and the problem is that once made, they are hard to put right. But the answer to that isn't *no* cosmetic surgery—it's *better* cosmetic surgery, more finely tuned lasers, more skilled technicians. The key has to be to take the time and trouble to find surgeons with a good track record. As more and more women who have had "work" done begin to speak out and tell their friends the good news, it will become easier and easier for those who are nervous to hear at first hand about who is good and who is not.

As to those who claim that cosmetic surgery is undignified and that they themselves would never do anything quite so drastic, when you take a good look at them they nearly always turn out to be twentysomething beauties who haven't the faintest idea of what it feels like to look in the mirror day after day and see one's reflection gradually going to pot. Just wait, I long to say to them, and see if you're quite so adamant when your own looks begin to fade. Read Nora Ephron's rail against the trials and tribulations of growing older and those who are either male or gloriously young will begin to get some idea that getting older, as Gore Vidal once put it, "isn't for sissies." But praise be, these days there are things—highly technical, skillful, successful things—that can be done and for that I think we should all be duly grateful.

But—and here I cannot stress this enough—it is absolutely key that you get the best surgeon you can. The difference between fine work and bad work is the difference between happiness and deep regret. Ask around among your friends. If you hear of a good plastic surgeon, ask to see before and after pictures.

I asked Mr. Barry Jones, plastic surgeon to any number of grateful women (who mostly keep deathly quiet about it) as well as, more importantly, to any number of desperately sick children and cancer patients, about the key questions that you should always ask your plastic surgeon before you embark on a face-lift. This was his advice.

Questions to Ask Your Plastic Surgeon

1. Are you on the American Board of Plastic Surgeons specialist register as a plastic surgeon?

2. Where did you train in plastic surgery, and when did you qualify?

3. Do you have privileges to conduct this procedure at a hospital or hospitals and, if so, where?

4. Are you a member of the American Society of Plastic Surgery (ASPS), the International Society of Aesthetic Plastic Surgeons (ISAPS), or the European Association of Plastic Surgeons (EURAPS)?

5. Do you have a specialist interest and, if so, can I reference any of your publications in peer-reviewed journals (e.g., *Plastic and Reconstructive Surgery* or *The American Journal of Cosmetic Surgery*) that would reflect it?

6. Having explained to you what I would like to achieve, is there a procedure that you would recommend?

7. What scarring can I expect?

8. How much swelling and/or bruising will there be?

9. How much pain might I expect?

10. How long need I stay in the hospital?

11. How long will it be before I can return to normal activities?

12. What complications may occur and what is their frequency?

13. How many of these operations do you do each year?

14. Which hospital do you operate at?

15. Does this procedure involve general anesthesia or sedation? If so, who is your anesthetist, and may I see a copy of their CV?

16. How much does it cost, and what exactly does that cover?

HEALTH

I'm not a medic, but I have learned a few things over the years. When I'm slimmer, I feel better and, of course, I look better. It's a bit of a struggle (no, I lie; it's a titanic struggle) for me because I'm only five feet two inches tall, and I have an underactive thyroid, and I love cooking, and I like wine, and I like eating with family and friends. And if you live in a city, as I do, a lot of your pleasures are sedentary—eating out, theaters, music—and writing, as I've always complained, is a very fattening occupation.

But losing weight isn't complicated. Although we all know what to do (eat sensibly and exercise more), sometimes we could do with a bit of help. For instance, I've never been to the Mayr Clinic (Dellach, Marie Worth on Lake Worth, Carinthia, Austria; +43 4273 2511; www.360travel.co.uk/mayr) but intend to one day. Everybody I know who has been has said it was as tough as Hades but paid off in spades.

How to Detox and Love It

I detoxed by mistake. I'd heard that in:spa was a fun place to go. Now, for those who haven't come across this fine institution in:spa is a newish company that has no fixed abode. It rents suitably big and sumptuous houses in delectable locations (such as Morocco, Ibiza, and Seville) and then brings the whole panoply of cooks, trainers, yoga teachers, masseurs and masseuses and nutritionists and all the rest to attend to all its customers' needs. Furthermore, I'd heard that they were running a week at Trasierra, Charlotte Scott's beautiful finca just outside Seville, with lots of pampering, massages, some lovely walks through the olive groves, exercise, and great healthy food. It sounded divine, so the husband and I went. *But* I hadn't read the small print.

It wasn't until we got there that we discovered that for the entire week there was to be no wheat, no dairy, no tea, no coffee, no alcohol, no red meat. I blanched at the news, but what I discovered was that it's *only* the compulsory removal of these things that makes the detox process—relatively—easy. We had no choice. The in:spa team made it fun and we had one of the most rewarding weeks of our lives. I don't think I lost as much weight as I would have liked (or thought I deserved), but I felt wonderfully well at the end of it and, for those who needed to get their eating and exercise on track, it was very educative (in the enjoyable sense of that word). For instance, one guest was a highly intelligent, high-earning girl who was really seriously overweight. (She didn't think she had a weight "ishoo" until she started losing it, which was when she realized how wonderful that made her feel.) However, she had no idea that avocados, while brilliantly nutritious, were laden with calories and should be eaten in small portions.

Everybody left at the end of the week with clearer skins, brighter eyes, and a great determination to take more exercise. I couldn't recommend it more highly.

In:spa takes its nutritionists, personal trainers, yoga teachers et al., to a series of divine locations, whether Ibiza, mainland Spain, or Marrakesh. Call them at +44 845 458 0723 for details or visit www.inspa-retreats.com to make a reservation.

The fundamentals behind detoxing are simple: to rid the body of the overload of toxins (alcohol, caffeine, and tannin, to name but a few) with which most of us assault it daily. It can easily—if you've got the willpower—be done at home. Everybody who tries it feel energized and cleansed afterwards. It usually involves a twenty-four-hour fast—nothing but water—

followed by some two weeks or so of nothing but fruit juices, herbal teas, and fruit and vegetables. Clearer eyes, cleaner livers, and much-increased energy are the usual benefits.

So You Want to Be Fitter?

> *Running is the best and, I think,*
> *the only cure for depression.*
> —LINDA RONSTADT

Taking exercise is the key to a healthy life and—more of an incentive perhaps to the vain among us—it's also key to keeping in reasonable shape. You don't want to become so overweight that you put your health at risk and you can't do the things you enjoy. So join a gym, get a personal trainer, take up tennis, ballroom dancing, cycling, swimming, or yoga—anything so long as it gets you moving. The trick is to find something you like as otherwise you won't stick with it. We all know by now—don't we?—that exercise releases chemicals called endorphins, which reduce feelings of anxiety and depression. It also makes you feel more alert and better able to cope with stress. You don't need to go overboard, although it can become awfully addictive: when some years ago my husband and I found ourselves running around the local pond late at night after the opera, I realized things had got out of hand. You should really aim for a minimum of thirty minutes a day doing something that makes you breathe slightly harder and feel slightly warmer than usual.

I happen to love both tennis and skiing. I play tennis with my husband and friends—not as often as I'd like but enough to keep me in reasonable shape. Skiing is trickier. My erstwhile skiing companions are all beginning to get "knees" or other ailments, and anyway it was never possible to do it for more than a couple of weeks a year.

I haven't found a gym near enough to me that I really like, so my solution—I know, I know, it's spoiling—is a personal trainer. Twice a week I have the wonderful Niki Day, and although it seems like an indulgence (when I tell my friends "she takes me for a walk, like a dog," they fall about laughing), it does get me out. She gets my heart rate up and makes me jog and stretch, and since I've paid for it I make a point of never missing a session.

There are personal trainers in every corner of the country, and if it's the only thing that makes you exercise, it's worth every penny. If you can discipline yourself to exercise on your own, well done—keep it up, and think of all the money you save.

So You Want to Be Thinner?

If you can't lose weight on your own (as I say, it is—relatively—simple: eat fewer fats, carbs, and sugar, and exercise more), professional help may be the answer. A year or so ago (in order to write a feature) I consulted Dr. Clark, an Edinburgh man who came to be interested in nutrition via his specialty in diabetes. He discovered that by controlling patients' diets, he could lower their insulin levels as a result of which their weight usually fell too. He's not primarily in business to help people lose weight—he's there to help them be healthy, and the process of eating healthily usually results in their losing weight. His regime normally reduces the so-called bad fats in the blood as well.

Dr. Clark started off by ordering a blood test to see just where everything was—thyroid, cholesterol, insulin, and all the other vital factors. "Everybody's biochemical profile is different. I've had very slim women come to me who have terrible biochemical profiles because they're, in effect, starving themselves of nourishment."

The principal weapon in the healthy diet is lowering insulin levels. Counting calories, he says, isn't what matters. It is much, much more important to reduce the intake of refined carbohydrates. They stimulate the production of insulin and it's insulin that converts those carbohydrates into fat. Those who are overweight often become locked into a vicious circle in which the refined carbohydrates that they eat mean that they manufacture more insulin, which in turn increases the desire for more carbohydrates.

I was given a diet sheet that was simple to say the least. I had to cut out all refined carbohydrates (cakes, biscuits, bread, pasta, rice); eat plenty of lean protein and lots of vegetables ("This is not a low carbohydrate diet," he points out. "It's high in carbohydrates, but the unrefined ones that are mostly found in vegetables"); cut out saturated fats; go easy on the alcohol (a glass or two a day of red wine); and that's it. It is, of course, our old friend the low-GI diet, fine-tuned to meet my individual needs after Dr. Clark had studied the blood test results.

I can tell you that it works, and it isn't onerous. When I followed it conscientiously, I went down from 143 pounds to 126 pounds. My insulin levels fell by 49 percent, my triglycerides by 18 percent and my LDL (low-density lipoproteins) by 10 percent, while the HDL (high-density lipoproteins—the so-called good fats) were up by 10 percent. I found it enormously helpful knowing that somebody would be checking my weight every other week. As the hand reached for the occasional chocolate, it would be stayed by the knowledge that the evidence would be all too easily spotted by Dr. Clark. His practice is at 14 Devonshire Place, London W1G 6HX. Call +44 20 7935 0640 for an appointment.

If you find it difficult to control your weight consider consulting a proper nutritionist. Oz Garcia's Longevity Lounge at 10 West Seventy-fourth Street, New York 10023; 212-579-9136, is a wonderful (if expensive) resource—he is responsible for helping Hilary Swank achieve her marvelous shape and fitness, but he's also helped countless others who aren't so famous. The thing about professional help is that by having your blood checked, all the various factors (cholesterols good and bad, insulin levels and all the rest) are monitored and knowing that you have to go back and all will be revealed keeps you on the straight and narrow.

> *If you have formed the habit of checking on every*
> *new diet that comes along, you will find that,*
> *mercifully, they all blur together, leaving you with*
> *only one definite piece of information:*
> *french–fried potatoes are out.*
>
> —JEAN KERR, WRITER

MASSAGE

If you thought massage was a delicious, optional extra, think again. Massage is seriously good for your health—and the older you get, the more you need it. According to Oz Garcia, of the brilliant Longevity Lounge, once you hit your fifties you should, if possible, have two massages a month. He says it keeps the muscles flexible, the toxins at bay, helps along a sluggish lymphatic system and prevents the build-up of knots of tension in necks and backs. In London, Dr. Ali, who treats many famous Brits, thinks that massaging the neck and shoulder area helps the functions of the pituitary gland (the headquarters of hormone control) by improving blood flow to the brain and he, too, thinks that twice a month is about right.

There are good masseurs/masseuses in many places and it may take time to find one near where you live. I like Pure Massage (3–5 Vanston Place, London SW6 1AY; +44 20 7381 8100; www.puremassage.com), which is in an unfashionable part of Fulham but it is sweet and clean, and has lovely spacious and calming treatment rooms. Although it has no grand pretensions, it has a serious purpose. Its founders, Beata Aleksandrowicz and Jean-Marc Delacourt, decided to concentrate solely on massage. To simplify the matter, they offer a small range of clear-cut options, all of which aim to be beneficial to health and well-being; they are not merely pampering, though they are that too. Beata offers seven different sorts of massage, most of which are a flexible combination of Thai massage, Swedish massage, and Indian head massage, using all the acupressure points, and which she has adapted to suit almost all clients. She uses massage to help with back problems; with migraines (often, says Beata, caused by strain and tension in the back); to relieve stress and tension, particularly in the neck and back; to help with lymphatic drainage, which keeps the immune system in good order; and to keep the joints and muscles flexible.

Like my friend, Oz Garcia, she believes that a one-off massage is fine, and better than nothing, but for optimum results you should go regularly and then see the difference it makes. "Each time you come back, the practitioner can go deeper into the muscle tissue, and you can release more toxins."

If you can't get to Pure Massage there are organizations everywhere, as well as independent masseuses who will come to your house. Go Massage (888-506-2772 and at www.gomassage .com) will send trained masseurs to you anywhere in the United States. New York Massage Company (212-427-8175 and at www.nymassage.com) will also send masseurs to addresses in the New York City area.

SCENT

A woman smells well when she smells of nothing.
—PLAUTUS (250–184 BCE),
ROMAN PLAYWRIGHT

Looking good is also about another very important intangible: scent. It is so fundamental to how I feel about myself that I can't imagine life without it.

I'm not ashamed to say that I'm a scent snob. I love the classic, complex, subtle scents of the great French houses— Caron, Guerlain, Nina Ricci, Dior, Creed, Chanel. I hate the cheap chemical smells, the harsh and strident concoctions that abound today. And, since I might as well make my prejudices clear, I personally can't bear most florals (though I make an exception for Guerlain's L'Heure Bleue) but I recognize that some of them are finely made and are some people's lifelong passion. The raison d'être of a fine scent is to reawaken a transitory, half-remembered world where memory and nostalgia, misty hopes and dreams all intermingle. The world it nudges into being should be rich and complex, haunting and insubstantial, but redolent with possibility, sensuality, and desire. I like scents to remind me of satins and furs and boxes at the opera, and dancing the night away, and falling in love, and all the things I cherish in life. In my experience, it's only the great classic scents that can do this.

Roja Dove, Professeur des Parfums and *éminence grise* of the perfume industry in the U.K., thinks scent "should be all about hedonism, indulgence, utter luxuriousness," which is why his Haute Parfumerie on the fifth floor at Harrods is one of the world's best places to learn about scent. There you will find not only the world's finest scents but some that are stocked by nobody else. "I've allowed my whimsies full rein in my

Haute Parfumerie," says Roja, "and haven't allowed commercial considerations to influence me one jot."

If you have one great signature scent that you love, the best way to wear it is to buy both the eau de toilette (80 percent of what you apply at eight A.M. will have dissipated by noon) and the parfum (50 percent will stay on the skin for twenty-four hours). Combine four or five pumps of the eau de toilette with a touch of perfume on the wrist, inside the dip of the collarbone, behind the knee and behind the neck.

☞ *Roja Dove says it is essential to wipe the parfum stopper after you've used it with a square of silk, as otherwise the oil from your body along with dead skin cells will contaminate the scent.*

Finally, there's the matter of the custom scent—one made especially for you, which I have never tried. This can be inordinately expensive (usually from $2,000, while if you want the master himself, Roja Dove, it'll cost you about $40,000) and my hunch is that it isn't worth it. There really are gorgeous scents around, some of them not worn by all and sundry, and to pay all that money and risk finding you don't like the result—it scarcely bears thinking about. I think the risk is too high.

Finally there is the matter of price. Really great scents aren't cheap. If you can't afford good ones it is better to wear nothing and do as master hotelier Gordon Campbell Grey does, simply smell divinely of nothing but fresh soap.

☞ *Not many women seem to know that the sun and scent combine to cause nasty pigmentation. Keep scent for when you're indoors.*

Perfumes can be divided into three main categories:

Florals: this is the largest and most varied category, ranging from simple florals (Diorissimo by Dior or Fracas by Robert Piguet) to big mixed bouquets (L'Heure Bleue by Guerlain or

L'Air du Temps by Nina Ricci). The aldehydic florals (Lanvin's Arpège or Chanel's No. 5) shimmer and sparkle while others (Vent Vert by Balmain or Truly by Stephen Burlingham) are crisp and fresh. All will have a sweetness that people either love or can't stand.

Florals are most liked by those of a happy, uncomplicated disposition, for whom every day is a sunny day.

Chypres: these are based around oak moss aided by cedar wood, vetiver, and patchouli, counterpointed by hesperidic (citrus) notes. Chypres have a dryness about them and are the most understated, pared-down formulas, which gives them their elegance and sophistication. These are the perfumery equivalent of a plain black evening gown from Valentino or a plain navy dress by Jean Muir. In other words, they take confidence to wear and are not for the fainthearted. Among the great chypres are Mitsouko by Guerlain, Tabac Blond by Caron, Farouche by Nina Ricci, Cabochard by Grès, La Perla by La Perla, Miss Dior by Dior, and Femme by Rochas.

Chypres are mostly chosen by strong-minded women who tend to see life in black-and-white terms, who know their own minds. If you're a minimalist at heart, then chypres are for you.

Orientals: these are based around vanilla (a psychogenic aphrodisiac that not only enhances pleasure for the wearer but has a very specific effect on others), sandalwood, gum resins from trees, and tonquin musk (from the tonka bean). They're rather hedonistic and self-indulgent—when they're good, they're wonderful, but when they're bad, they can be cloying and pervasive, verging on the vulgar. The great orientals are Shalimar by Guerlain, Opium by Yves Saint Laurent, Must de Cartier, French Can Can by Caron, Bal à Versailles by Jean Desprez, Vol de Nuit by Guerlain, and Nuit de Noël by Caron.

They are worn by women who are larger than life and generally like to be noticed. These are women who know how to use their femininity to their own advantage and know exactly which shade of lipstick, height of heel, and length of hem suits them best.

Roja Dove's Guide to Choosing Scent

1. Allow yourself time. It could be the start of a lifelong love affair.

2. Choose your store carefully. Those that have separate counters for every perfume house are not the best environments for this particular exercise. Go to a specialist shop (see page 152) where there is somebody who cares passionately about scent.

3. Go wearing no scent but armed with a pen and pad to note names.

4. Smell some florals, chypres, and orientals, and by a process of elimination, decide which group pleases you most. Most testers are marked on the back with the words "fleuri" or "florale" (indicating florals), "chypres" and either "orientale" or "amber."

5. Think of the scent strips as hangers for clothes. Only when you put on the clothes (scent) will you really know whether it suits you but in the meantime you can judge quite a lot while it is still on the hanger (scent strip). Take about five or six strips to test the different scents. Don't smell them right away. Walk away and then smell them two at a time, one and then the other. Ask yourself which of the two you prefer and put aside the one you like least. Then compare your preferred strip with another and again discard the one you like least. You will soon come to the one or two you like best. Keeping these, go and sit somewhere quiet to compare and contrast. When you decide which one you like best, spray it on your wrists (do *not* rub it in), a little bit on the collarbone and a mist around your hair. Then leave the store and go home. "Just like a lover, you'll only know whether

the love affair will last if you spend the night together, so take some home. Otherwise you could end up with a *mésalliance.*" If you still love the scent the next day, go and buy some. Lastly, you shouldn't really just "like it" either—you should fall madly, passionately in love.

Shops for Scent Around the World

NEW YORK

Aedes De Venustas (9 Christopher Street, New York 10014; 212-206-8674; www.aedes.com) sells all the most divine little niche perfumes (from Carthusia, Creed, Etro, Cote Bastide, and a particularly gorgeous chypre, limited edition Eau de Parfum by Molinard) as well as some of its own lines. Gorgeous things for the home and the bath are to be found as well. Everything comes in its own beautiful black boxes. A jewel of a shop, and it sells online.

Bond No. 9 (9 Bond Street, New York 10012; 212-228-1732; www.bondno9.com)—another lovely little niche shop with some of its own line of fragrances, all dedicated to different areas of New York (Broadway, Wall Street, and so on).

Le Labo (233 Elizabeth Street, New York 10012; 212-219-2230; www.lelabofragrances.com) is a lovely niche brand, with little-known perfumes by Fabrice Penot and Eddie Roschi (who used to be at Giorgio Armani fragrances). They blend essential oils and alcohol and water when you buy them and they sometimes create niche lines for a particular city (Dallas, Paris).

Perfumania (755 Broadway, New York 10003; 212-979-7674; www.perfumania.com)—just one of some seven branches, all specializing in niche perfumes as well as most popular brands.

My Favorite Scents

Guerlain's Shalimar used to be my all-time favorite, but now they seem to have changed the
composition (partly, as I understand it, because
of European Union rules and partly because of
the difficulty and expense of getting some of the
rare ingredients) and now I find it too heavy and
unsubtle. I still love Guerlain's Jicky, Vol de Nuit,
L'Heure Bleue, and Mitsouko.

- Quadrille by Balenciaga (a great classic now
  revived).
- Narcisse Noir (a favorite of the Ballets
  Russes), and Tabac Blond, a wonderfully sensuous chypre, both by Caron.
- Ormonde by Ormonde Jayne.
- Ambre Soie (rich, dark, and warm, with hints
  of cinnamon, cloves, and Chinese ginger),
  and Bois d'Encens, both by Armani Privé,
  and only to be found in the best Giorgio Armani boutiques.
- Bel Ami by Hermès.
- Ambre Sultan by Serge Lutens.
- Feminite du Bois by Shiseido.
- Shocking by Schiaparelli, because it's the first
  scent my father ever gave me. It brings back
  happy days in Aldeburgh and walking along
  the estuary in the long summer evenings.
- Yerbamate and Spezie by Lorenzo Villoresi.

In summer or on vacation I often wear something
lighter. Diptyque's Philosykos smells divinely,
subtly of fig. I also love Jo Malone's Ginger and
Nutmeg.

LONDON

Roja Dove's Haute Parfumerie on the fifth floor at Harrods, 87–135 Brompton Road, London SW1X 7XL (+44 20 7897 8797), or one of the three Roja Dove perfumeries in House of Fraser stores.

L'Artisan Parfumeur, 17 Cale Street, London SW3 3QR (+44 20 7352 4196), is a delightful shop with lots of small niche perfumes.

Les Senteurs, 71 Elizabeth Street, London SW1W 9PJ (+44 20 7730 2322). James Craven has a passion for scent and is seriously knowledgeable. The shop also has a brilliant catalogue with great descriptions of the perfumes it carries and will send out up to six little sample phials at £2.50 ($5) a phial.

Ormonde Jayne, the Royal Arcade, 28 Old Bond Street, London W15 451 (+44 207 499 1100). Linda Pilkington is a relatively new perfumer on the block but her products are lovely. She's made her name by using lesser-known ingredients that give her perfumes a certain exoticism. Fans are mad for her grapefruit candles and I love her Ormonde fragrance. Her bath oils are gorgeous, too.

PARIS

There are some gorgeous places to visit in Paris.

Chanel is best known for Chanel No. 5 (with Marilyn Monroe declaring it was all she wore to bed, how could it fail?) but not everybody knows that if you go to its boutiques (and there isn't a better one than Boutique Chanel, 31 rue Cambon, Paris 75001; +33 1 42 86 26 00, where Coco herself held court), you can buy some very special scents that aren't sold anywhere else. Cuir de Russie is my favorite, but I also like Bois des Iles and No. 22, while Gardenia is for those who are into florals. Six more special, boutique-only scents have just been launched, known as Les Exclusifs, and all by Jacques Polge, Chanel's "nose." Worth investigating.

Serge Lutens was for years the creative director of Shiseido and he helped develop many of its scents, in particular the gorgeous Feminite du Bois. Now he has his own line, all of which are divine, though as perfume is such a personal thing, you'll love some more than others. Me, I love most of them but particularly Borneo 1834 and Ambre Sultan. Go to his jewel of a shop, Les Salons du Palais Royal Shiseido, Jardins du Palais Royal, 142 Galérie de Valois, Paris 75001; +33 1 49 27 09 09, and leave yourself time to try them all.

Frédéric Malle (Editions de Parfums Frédéric Malle, 37 rue de Grenelle, Paris 75007; +33 1 42 22 76 40), whose grandfather founded Parfums Christian Dior, has some wonderful perfumes, including Le Parfum de Thérèse. It was made by the great "nose" Edmond Roudnitska for his wife during the 1960s and he gave Frédéric Malle the right to make it after his death. It's lush and languid and has a cult following.

La Maison de Guerlain, 68 avenue des Champs Elysées, Paris 75008; +33 1 45 62 11 21, is a gorgeous boutique that has all the glamour one expects of the grandest of all parfumiers. Here you can not only try all the greats but there's a series of boutique-only experiences and scents that "vaut le détour."

Annick Goutal, 14 rue de Castiglione, Paris 75001; +33 1 42 60 52 82.

FLORENCE

Lorenzo Villoresi, Via de' Bardi 14, Florence 50125 is for my money one of the greatest living perfumers, but you must make an appointment to visit—call +39 55 2341 187 or info@lorenzo villoresi.it. Villoresi is from an old Florentine family and in his laboratory at the top of a medieval palazzetto overlooking the

Arno, he mixes up wonderfully complex and exotic perfumes. These capture the smell of cut grass, the Mediterranean (sage, rosemary, myrtle, thyme), tobacco, and wild poppy, among many others. There are divine room candles and potpourris too. Some are available in the U.S. (at Lafco NY, with locations in New York and Los Angeles), but if you're in Florence you'd be foolish not to visit his little atelier. He will also make you a custom scent in about two hours for $2,000, which is infinitely cheaper than anybody else.

Farmaceutica di Santa Maria Novella, Via della Scala 16, Florence 50123; +39 55 216 276, is one of the world's oldest pharmacies or herbalists, dating from 1612, with divine soaps—the pomegranate especially—lotions, colognes, and powders. It's an experience just to see the shop even if you buy nothing.

There are also some fabulous Web sites for those who love niche, complex, beautiful perfumes— **www.beautyhabit.com** and **www.mimifroufrou.com/ scentedsalamander**, which will keep you up to date with new perfume launches and gives its own highly opinionated reviews and musings on fragrant subjects.

THREE

love,

marriage,

and

happiness

Love

Speak to me of love; I thirst for it.

—ALEXANDER PUSHKIN TO
ANNA PETROVNA KERN, SEPTEMBER 22, 1825

Most of us need love in our lives in order to feel alive, let alone happy. We need to love as well as to be loved, and if we can achieve both we are immeasurably blessed. For most of us it is the one true essential, the basis of our lives. But there are so many different kinds of love and different ways of loving. There's nothing like the adrenalin rush of "being in love," which is, of course, a kind of madness, an intoxication that can turn out to be a fatal attraction that causes days, months, even years of grief . . . or it can be the stepping stone to a more grounded, enduring sort of love that leads to a lifelong marriage. But love was ever a mystery. It works in deep, unknown ways and there are no certain answers to any of the big questions: "Why does he not love me anymore?" "Why has he/she left me?" Love changes—indeed, it must change if it is to endure—and it can take many forms.

How can we tell real, enduring love from its more intoxicating cousin, infatuation? That's the big question. If we knew *that,* the world wouldn't be littered with broken hearts and failed relationships, and half the world's literature would never have been written. But just as there are no pat answers, there are no formulaic rules. And there is comfort to be found in the fact that pain and heartbreak are the other side of caring, and the more you care, the more it hurts. This applies to any form of love. Every mother will tell you that from the moment her child is born, whole new acres of possible suffering—as well as joy, of course—are opened up.

But for those for whom long-lasting love has never happened, who have been widowed or divorced, who for one reason or another find themselves alone, there are all sorts of other ways of loving. There are children and godchildren to love, there are mothers and fathers, brothers and sisters, friends and the big wide world to channel all that love into.

All I know is that love comes out of the blue, sometimes when you least expect it, and that the key is not necessarily to go looking for it but to keep your mind and heart wide open to the larger horizon. Those who keep looking outwards, who can find it in themselves to reach out to what life brings them, who feel that sense of possibility in the air, are those to whom things happen.

Marriage

God grant me the serenity to accept the things
I cannot change, the courage to change the things
that I can, and the wisdom to know the difference.
—Reinhold Niebuhr, "The Serenity Prayer"

We have only to look around us to see that there is no blueprint for marriage. Every marriage is different. We see (a few) so-called traditional wives who prefer to defer to their husbands, who are happy for them to do most of the earning and most of the decision-making, and for the two people in that particular marriage it seems to work. And then we know of other people who would find it so stifling and claustrophobic that one or other would have run away screaming into the night after just a few months.

Other couples evolve completely different sort of partnerships. Sometimes the woman is an equal partner financially and plays a proactive role in all the major decisions involving the family. In others, she may sometimes be the sole earner and the couple has mutually decided that it suits their circumstances best for the husband to play what used conventionally to be the female role—the caregiver, the domestic rock, and the financially dependent partner. There are as many psychological and practical arrangements as there are couples. All we know is that if there is a formula, nobody's found it yet.

Good marriages are all about "fit," about the degree to which each partner's hopes, expectations, talents, and dreams can be allowed to grow and flourish—and, of course, they are also about love. At first sight the institution doesn't seem to be in the most robust health. Most of us have only to think about our close and immediate circles of family and friends to see divorce on a scale that would have been thought socially unacceptable for our parents' generation. I myself grew up with divorced parents in the South Africa of the 1940s and 1950s, and it always made me feel a child apart, for I was for many years the only child I knew whose living parents were no longer married. Today, however, divorce is commonplace.

The statistics bear this out. Two out of five marriages at the moment are doomed to end in divorce—though to look on the bright side that means that three out of five survive. Who would have thought, fifty years ago, that three out of four of the queen of England's children would be divorced? Add to this the number of people who aren't bothering to get married at all, and the numbers of children born to single women or women who are in relationships with "partners," and it appears that the institution of marriage is in deep trouble.

In my close circle, one of my dearest friends tells me that her children—attractive, clever, in their thirties with great careers—aren't even considering marriage for, as they remind her, "You and Daddy have seven marriages between you [which she has to admit is true], and we don't know many people who have stayed married, so we can't quite see the point."

One of the things that has changed is that in the practical sense women don't need a man in the way they used to. The old joke that "Marriage was the price men paid for sex while sex was the price women paid for marriage" seems so archaic now as to belong to another world. Women can earn their own livings, have a perfectly satisfying social life, enjoy the pleasures of sex and even have children without tying the knot. IVF, sperm banks, financial independence, and multiple fluid relationships—all things unthinkable merely forty years ago— have played their part in changing the way we relate to our friends, our families, and our children.

I recently read of a young woman who, feeling that her biological clock was beginning to tick, decided that while she was perfectly resigned to not having a man in her life, she could not reconcile herself to life without a child. In years gone by this would have been an insoluble dilemma. No more. She found no fewer than three different men who were only too delighted to meet her need for an arm's-length, sanitized form of parenthood: a young gay man; a much older, married, childless man; and a single straight man of her own age. Problem—at one level—solved.

It seems so flexible, so modern, but I have my doubts as to how deeply these new arrangements meet the psychological and practical needs of either men or women, let alone the children. For this loosening of old attitudes has had a dramatic effect on the plight of children. In the United States some 40 percent of children are currently born out of wedlock, and while the phrase itself may seem harsh and out of date, the reality is that most children flourish best in what we have learned to call the family. It is obvious that loving care—and this clearly *can* be provided by loving parents who are not married—is what children need to grow into healthy, well-adjusted human beings who have self-respect and respect for others. When you read the stories behind the juvies that we have created today, nearly every one is a poignant human tragedy, of children who have not been loved and nurtured, who live with mothers who may have several children by various vanished fathers, who seem not to know how to be proper wives or mothers. The jails are full of people who come from dysfunctional families who were not mostly, or even usually, born bad but who were not given that essential start in life, that age-old security that only love and care, which seems best provided by a mother and a father who are married to each other, can provide. This loosening of ties and lack of social boundaries has led to too many men and women having children for which they don't provide proper, stable homes.

It would be wrong to ignore the upside—women no longer need allow themselves to be bullied and marginalized; their talents need no longer be neglected; they have paths to professional fulfillment and economic freedom; there is a chance for greater honesty in relationships—but we also see that more and more women at least are beginning to sense that professional success and economic freedom often come at a great price. We see women who are made lonely by their freedom, their lack of ties, their financial independence. I remember well being at a professional meeting where there were some highly successful women around the table. Somebody mentioned that one of our previous colleagues had got married and had retired to be a mother of three in the country. One of the most successful of all the women said with a voice full of envy, "Oh, wow . . . " And it rapidly became clear that for the farmhouse, the kids, the dogs in the back of the car, the husband, the busy family life, she'd give it all up tomorrow. Underneath she felt a deep longing that was something she couldn't help, an old biological recognition of the need to bond, of one man to commit to one woman, and to create a safe haven for each other and their children. A longing, too, to be, as my friend Sandy Boler, the former editor of *Brides* (U.K.) magazine, put it, "to be safely gathered in"—something that marriage in its best and most reassuring form can do.

Which is possibly why I detect in the air, in the zeitgeist, something of a seismic backlash. Women—and marriage has always been more in a woman's interest than a man's—have come to see that too much insistence on egalitarianism hasn't brought them the dreamed-of utopia. Insisting that a man who works long hours also does his share of the cooking and the diaper changing while his wife whirls around with her own career may succeed in bringing about help with the chores, but it doesn't often lead to that woman being deeply loved. An insistence on strict division of labor seems to me to smack of minding more about "one's rights" than any notion of real love. It would, surely, often be better to do rather more than your share of the housework and have a happy home and a husband who loves you.

You now see high-earning alpha women who seem to be indulging in what one commentator called "competitive breeding": for instance, those two fantastically high-earning titans of the finance industry, Nicola Horlick (with six children) and Helena Morrissey (with seven) are creating and building very large families, as if to compensate for the masculine world in which they spend their days. You sense a kind of yearning for the sort of domestic dreams and certainties that were the norm some forty or fifty years ago, but which these days have gotten lost in dreams of breaking through glass ceilings and forging free and independent lives.

The *New York Times* columnist Maureen Dowd put it beautifully when she wrote: "Five years ago, you would often hear high-powered women fantasize that they would love a Wife, somebody to do the shopping, cooking, carpooling, so they could focus on work. Now the fantasy is more retro: They just want to be that Wife."

Those of us who are married know that marriage isn't always easy—though, heaven knows, it's always seemed to me so much nicer than the alternative. Since many of us are lucky enough to live much longer than primitive man was privileged to do, we know that long-lasting marriages—some of forty, fifty, and even sixty years—have strains and stresses of their own, but it is hard to think of a better institution for meeting our deepest human needs.

Almost no marriage is perfect (and, interestingly, if it is, the children often suffer quite badly—remember writer Alice Thomas Ellis's quip that "Men love women, women love children and children love their hamsters"), but nobody has yet come up with a better way to meet our most profound longings. De facto marriage—a serious commitment between a man and a woman, whether blessed by a priest or not—reaches far back into antiquity. It evolved because it was what men, women and their children required if society was to be whole and sane. A really good marriage should, most psychologists think, meet three crucial needs: the longing for real emotional intimacy; the need for a sense of self-worth; and a greater possibility of both partners fulfilling their goals in life.

But marriage is an ever-evolving institution. Modern ones have had to adapt and change. Many women now earn more than their spouses. The lucky, well-adjusted spouses are happy and grateful for it, but the less secure seem to require even more nurturing, so that the working wife is locked into a syndrome where the harder she works, and the more money she brings in, the more she has to show on the home front that she isn't neglecting her domestic skills and that he isn't a "house husband." Where both spouses are highly successful and there are children, something has to give if the marriage *and* the children are to be nurtured—and if it isn't the woman who is prepared to give up some of her high-flying years, then I see trouble ahead. It may not be fair, but what is the alternative?

Many marriages these days are second and third marriages, requiring a greater generosity of spirit, a real willingness to forgive, to put away past bitternesses, and an extra effort to make these multiple complex relationships work. Sometimes I'm astounded at the warmth and nobility with which some new relationships can be made to work if those involved bring a real desire to create something good out of what could be destructive chaos. I see stepchildren who love their stepparents and their stepsiblings; I see rejected wives moving on from their natural feelings of hurt and pain in order to ease the path for children and stepchildren. Of course you see the reverse as well—those who can never escape their feelings of injury and rejection, whose bitterness lives on, creating yet more difficulties for those around them. But they are the ones for whom there is usually no moving on, no different other life, which those who can put away their past suffering can sometimes find.

"Food and plenty of sex," says one high-flying wife, are the key to keeping a husband happy. If you keep both of those flowing, you can get away with a bit of neglect on other fronts. Whatever it takes, it seems to me that the rewards of having a husband or partner who loves you, who cares for his home and children, are worth cherishing. If swinging from the chandelier is what it takes, then do it—that's my view.

A Few Things I've Learned Along the Way

❧ Don't nag. It's not worth it. It's simpler and more conducive to a happy household to do whatever it is yourself.

❧ Concentrate on the things you love about him, not the things that drive you mad.

❧ Manners matter: politeness, kindness, tolerance, generosity of spirit.

❧ Try to think of things that please your other half: meals, books, adventures, small treats. All these are ways of showing love.

❧ Remember he has needs too.

❧ Don't harbor regrets or dwell on past hurts.

❧ Do your best to love his family—although some of them may be more lovable than others—and always welcome them to the house.

❧ You don't own the person you married. They are still entitled to some freedoms, to their own views and their own space. The best marriages provide a secure framework in which individuals can grow and flourish, not wither and diminish.

❧ It's worth making time to be together, so plan time together and little pleasures. It's particularly hard when there are small children, but grandparents or babysitters can be roped in. One couple who found that they were always so busy that they never had time to talk in a connected way made a date once a week to have lunch out—not a fancy lunch, just a simple diner lunch—and they found that they began to rediscover each other.

❧ Find things that you like to do together. Try to take an interest in his hobbies, friends and sports and in return he should try to take an interest in yours.

❧ Never run him down in public.

☞ The New Couple: Why the Old Rules Don't Work and What Does, *by Maurice Taylor and Seana McGee, is worth reading for all those troubled by the fast-changing dynamics of coupledom as well as for those who Taylor and McGee call the "scared singles." Check out www.newcouple.com.*

MONEY

We all know that money doesn't buy happiness—there are plenty of miserable millionaires and billionaires around to prove the point (though, as some trophy wife pointed out, it's a whole lot nicer to be miserable in comfort than in penury). But some money is, in my view, essential for self-respect. I've earned my own money since I was twenty and, though I have the most generous of husbands, I would never, ever like to have to ask for every penny I needed. In *A Room of One's Own,* Virginia Woolf came to the conclusion that if a woman was to write fiction (for which read: "do anything interesting or important at all"), a woman needed her own income and a room of her own. I would say that for all women, no matter what their status, it's important to contrive to have some—not necessarily a great deal—but some money of their own and to find something of their own space to be their own person. Who, after all, would want to be the other half of a "passenger," of somebody without a proper life or interests of their own?

A friend of mine who doesn't earn her own money (her husband earns plenty) jokes that she has compiled a "running away" fund out of the housekeeping expenses. She has no intention of running away—she loves her husband dearly—but she does like to know that she can. I understand completely. The idea here is that true relationships, the best relationships, are founded on a certain degree of independence, between two people who are properly whole in their own right. A friend who married a very rich—and very nice and wise—man was given $2 million on her wedding day by her new husband. He wanted to know, for his own happiness and satisfaction, that she was staying with him because she wanted to—not because she had to.

To be totally dependent on a man for money limits your freedom, no matter how kindly and generous the man. The same is true for men—a certain degree of economic security is essential to be really free. It's why men, instead of having "running away" funds, have what they like to call "fuck you" money. It enables them to be courageous in difficult situations, to walk away when they need to. So I feel that women, for their own sense of self-worth, should always find a way of having or earning money of their own. Even if it's a small part-time job, it at least means that if you're set on buying something that he doesn't like, you can spend your own money on it, and more importantly, when you buy him a present, you're paying for it. That apart, my view on work is that work (which doesn't necessarily have to be hugely financially rewarding) sustains you through many difficult times in life—it gives shape and meaning to your life, expands your knowledge and interests and sees you through periods of loneliness, bereavement, and heartache.

GETTING HELP

Many marriages—and relationships—run into difficulties. Some of them can be repaired and professional counseling can be an enormous help, not just to the man and wife but to any children involved as well. The American Association for Marriage and Family Therapy offers resources for finding a trained therapist in your community. Check out their Web site at www.therapistlocator.net, and you'll find a list of the standard problems that crop up in many marriages: "I've had an affair, how do I tell my partner?" or "My partner and I just don't seem to talk any more and it feels as if we've drifted apart," or "I can't seem to stop arguing with my partner, what can we do?" It helps to know that, whatever it is that is troubling you, marriage counselors will almost certainly have seen something like it before. You are not alone.

Others find help in psychotherapy, but here it is vital to make sure of the caliber of the therapist—the good ones are marvelous, the bad ones dangerous. Try to get recommendations from friends who might know of good ones through personal experience. Otherwise contact the National Board for Certified Counselors (www.counselorfind.org or 336-547-0607).

DIVORCE

Divorce is right up there as one of the most stressful events life can bring, being only less painful than the death of a child or somebody very close to you. Even the most amicable of divorces spreads ripples of pain well beyond the couple themselves—most of all to the children, if any, of the marriage. However, mothers, fathers, siblings, and friends will also feel the fallout.

On the other hand, some abusive or destructive relationships, or ones that are plain worn out, where neither side can muster any affection, tenderness or respect for the other, are clearly better ended. Calling time is sometimes the only way to a better future. These days, there are two pluses: at least it can be done without having to cast blame or exchange insults, and two, as people live longer and more healthily, many divorcees go on to make new and happy second (and even third and fourth) relationships.

Besides dealing with the emotional pain, there are legal and financial implications, as well as domestic arrangements, that have to be taken into account. Here the blessings of friendship really count. Talking to friends, feeling encircled by people who care, can ease the pain but nonetheless professional help is almost always needed.

> Organizations such as Woman's Divorce (www.womansdivorce.com) and the Smart Divorce (www.thesmartdivorce.com) are great sources of help. The Smart Divorce offers counseling, as well as advice on everything from where to go for legal help (it believes in promoting an approach to divorce that minimizes the financial, what it calls collaborative law as a new and more dignified approach to divorce) to how to find support groups.

WIDOWHOOD

This is usually another deeply painful life event, particularly for couples so closely bound that they can't ever envisage another partner. But, to be truthful, I have known some widows and widowers find a completely new lease on life as the patterns of an old way of life are thrown off and a fresh life beckons. How successfully people adapt and heal is often very dependent upon whether they still have work that is rewarding, whether they have nurtured friendships and have a warm close circle to call on, and how financially comfortable they are.

Since usually men die rather younger than women, it follows that there are rather more widows than widowers, which means that not all widows can hope to remarry. But full and rich lives can still be lived. Friendships, hobbies, travel, a warm and open heart that takes pleasure in small things, and an interest in other people, can all help to build a different sort of life.

Caring Connections is a nonreligious organization designed to help anybody who has been bereaved. This includes young people and parents of children who have died, but Cruse was originally set up with the aim of improving end-of-life care. It offers support in lots of ways, including one-to-one counseling. Contact Cruse via the Web site (www.crusebereavementcare.org.uk) or call the helpline (+44 844 477 9400).

www.widowsource.com provides support for those who are widowed or who have lost partners.

Friendship

Always anticipate your friends' needs,
never wait until they have to ask.
—Maria Huxley (wife of Aldous Huxley)

Nurture your friendships—they matter more than you can possibly imagine. Of all the things I most regret, it is perhaps working too much and not giving enough time to my friends. When you see the banana skins that lie await in life—the love affairs and marriages that go wrong, the illnesses that hit most of us at some time or another, and all the other more minor tragedies that make up life's great tapestry—it is friends and lovers who see you through. If you have them, you can cope with almost anything. And you also need friends to share good fortune with—it's pretty pointless enjoying the good times alone. We all hope not to be a friend of the Gore Vidal sort, he who once proclaimed: "For true happiness it is not enough to be successful oneself . . . one's friends must fail."

Friendship, though, needs maintenance. It means giving time and thought to our friends and, for many of us, absorbed as we are by our jobs and our families, it is hard to find time to do as much as we would like. It is perhaps one of the consolations of the empty-nest syndrome that as the children leave home, parents once again become more outgoing, able to renew old friendships and make new ones. Once again they find they have the sort of time that they haven't usually had since their twenties.

How do you keep friendships alive when you're having trouble juggling work and family and there's scarcely a free minute in the day? It's difficult, but there are ways. If friends are much the same age and at the same stage in life—whether single, what Bridget Jones called the "smug marrieds," bogged down by their children, coping with teenagers, or empty nesters—it makes it that much easier, for your interests are already aligned. Singles can go out clubbing (if that's their thing), see plays or form book clubs together. Later, as marriage and families come along, you can do things as married couples, and then get together as families for Sunday lunches and walks, softball games, tennis, whatever.

But the real way to show your friendship is to be there when times get tough and to help celebrate when there's a success. We all remember the friend who lifted the phone and offered to help when one of you lost a job, who visited the hospital when you were ill, who sent flowers or a letter when some disaster hit or there was something to celebrate.

One friend who lost her husband horribly early to cancer has never forgotten the woman friend who rang every day to begin with, and later on every week, to find out how she was, and to invite her over for dinner or to the movies.

Friends most particularly should be there when people they care about are ill. When my brother was ill and dying of cancer I discovered that some friends found the whole situation embarrassing. They didn't know what to say, so they said nothing. It wasn't that they didn't care but they didn't care enough to get over their embarrassment. Real friendship, in my view, should have meant minding more about my brother, whose predicament and suffering was real, than their own discomfort.

Another friend was bitterly hurt when one of her closest friends seemed to abandon her when she got breast cancer. When she saw her at a reception, the friend waved an airy hand and said, "Do call me if you need anything." That is *not* how you do it. You call, you visit, you write, you try to anticipate what might help. You take a meal over to the house, offer music to listen to or books to read. You might also think of the partner of the person who is ill, who often is having a tough time, too, but real friendship involves anticipating the need and trying to fill it—not waiting to be asked.

Friendship, in the end, is simple, if time-consuming. It means doing for your friends what you hope they'd do for you.

On Being a Daughter

There are so many phases to being a daughter, ranging from those early years when your mother is a golden goddess who can do no wrong (as my daughter once put it, "Mother, until I was about twelve, I thought you were perfect!") to the final later years when the person who once cared for us as children and young adults now needs to be cared for themselves. It's one of the most painful of all adjustments to make but the great thing is that there is now a great deal of help at hand.

Things to Do with the Elderly

❈ Take them to the movies once a week or re-create the experience at home—play a DVD, buy popcorn, make it fun.

❈ Get them books on tape to listen to or books in big type from the library. Contact Books Aloud (408-808-2613 and at www.booksaloud.org).

❈ Find an adult education class they'd like.

❈ Organize painting or photography classes—or anything else that interests them.

❈ Take them to a gallery or museum once a month.

❈ Start a book club with likeminded friends.

❈ You could start with your family doctor, who will be able to point you in the direction of district nurses, social workers, home care organizers and a bevy of other therapists, if they are deemed necessary.

❈ Your local library has a long list of agencies that can provide help, as well as useful pamphlets and leaflets.

❈ If you need advice on benefits and bureaucracy, try contacting the Citizen Information Center (800-333-4636), or 311 can nearly always guide you to other sorts of help.

❈ The National Council on Aging (www.ncoa.org), Eldercare Locator (their helpline is 800-677-1116 and at www.elder care.gov), Medicare Initiative (www.medicareinitiative.org) and Caring Connections (www.caringinfo.org) offer lots of advice.

❈ Remember, too, to get legal advice over tricky areas like disability, welfare, social security, and power of attorney. The latter must be sorted out while the elderly person is of sound mind—it is too late once they are no longer capable of making that decision.

❧ Caregiver Needed (919-673-4757 and at www.caregiver needed.com) can offer companions to read, guide, drive, and escort elderly people.

❧ But remember, caregivers themselves may need help too. Don't be afraid to ask for it and don't wear yourself out—that doesn't help anybody. If you are a caregiver, you might like to know that there is a support group near you: contact the National Family Caregivers Association (800-896-3650 and at www.nfcacares.org), and you will find a great deal of useful information on support services.

ON BEING A GRANDMOTHER

Where have all the grannies gone? I mean the genuine, original, 22-carat articles who wore black shawls and cameo brooches, sat in rocking chairs and smelled of camphor?

—KEITH WATERHOUSE, ENGLISH NOVELIST,
PLAYWRIGHT, AND COLUMNIST

Being a grandmother is wonderful—particularly when it comes, as it usually does these days, slightly later in life than it did in times gone by, so that by the time it happens, you are good and ready (I'm not sure I would have much liked being a "granny" in my forties). It is a great joy to find a succession of babies, toddlers, and slightly older children back in your life after the years in between that were bereft of the sweet sounds and smells of tiny children. I'm not as good a grandmother as I'd always dreamed of being. I always thought I'd be the doting kind and though I do dote—all five of them, as far as I'm concerned, can do no wrong—I'm too busy to be doing much of the apple-pie baking or the babysitting. And I'm not alone—

grannies all around us are trekking in the Himalayas, writing books or running companies, and so our children's generation is having to get used to the fact that the apple-cheeked, ever available, domestic granny is a long-gone stereotype. But that can have its upsides. All my grandsons have been promised that they will be taken to Africa when they turn ten, and since I'm just back from the first such expedition (to Botswana: such fun for me and, I hope, for him), I'm glowing at the moment with the memory of it all.

As I didn't have any proper grannies myself (my father's mother had fifteen children and I don't even know how many grandchildren, so I was simply one among a vast, undifferentiated horde; while my mother's mother was too hostile to my father to take much to his daughter), I aim to be the kind of granny that I wish I'd had.

I consider myself unbelievably lucky in both my son-in-law and daughter-in-law, who seem to welcome us whenever we are around and who never keep their children from us but want us to love and cherish them, as we do. Other grandparents, I know, are not so lucky and seeing their grandchildren sometimes seems fraught with difficulties. The straight facts of the matter are that once your children are married and have left the nest, there is a power shift: usually grandparents need their children and grandchildren rather more than the children need the grandparents. Which is why it seems not only wise but essential to try to make sure that there are no rifts or spats and also that you have a proper role to play and never become a mere encumbrance or a duty.

> *I can't be a grandmother. I'm too young.*
> *Grandmothers are old. They bake and they sew.*
> *I was at Woodstock! I pissed in the fields.*
> —Karen Buckman, *Parenthood*

How to Be a Good Grandmother

- Never forget that they're not your children. You've had your turn—now it's theirs.
- Never criticize anybody—son, daughter, in-laws, children. As far as you're concerned, they're all perfect.
- Offer advice only if it's asked for.
- Don't drop by all the time without being asked.
- Try to make visits fun, and think of interesting things to do with the grandchildren.
- Remember all birthdays and exam times, and always offer congratulations when they're due.
- Always respect the rules of your grandchildren's parents.
- If you see that they are in difficulties of any kind, don't criticize—offer help.
- Never show favoritism. You may have favorites (grandparents are only human), but keep them to yourself and let nobody guess.
- Never undermine the parents.
- Never be competitive with the other grandparents—it's not grown-up, and it's pointless.
- Try to be useful—and fun.
- Think of a role you can play that nobody else can.

Ten Things to Do with Grandchildren

1. Take a musical grandchild to a first concert, a ballet dancer to their first ballet, a sports-mad one to his first major-league game.

2. From time to time, take each one to something on their own where you can have a special time alone. Choose something that matches their interest.

3. Take one to see a couple (no more) of special pictures at a museum and talk to them about why they're special. Follow it up with sundaes at Serendipity 3, or your local equivalent.

4. When they reach a certain age, take them on a suitable unusual holiday (as I've already said, mine get taken to Africa for their tenth birthday)—to see the pyramids, to Paris, to Rome, the Victoria Falls, to a musical festival . . . whatever.

5. Just before Christmas take them to see Santa Claus at the North Pole. (www.santatripsonline.co.uk.)

6. Teach them some games—hearts, bridge, gin rummy, chess, poker, charades.

7. Teach them how to do something you're good at—such as cooking, gardening, tennis, riding, sailing, skiing.

8. Introduce them to books you've loved that you think they might like.

9. Take a teenage girl shopping for clothes (e.g., her first grown-up party dress), makeup, or for whatever interests her.

10. Plan a special overnight treat—such as a camping, riding, or sailing weekend, or teach them to fish in Yellowstone, the Chesapeake, or the Grand Canyon.

☞ *Two invaluable guides:* The Grandparents' Book *by Miriam Stoppard, published by Dorling Kindersley, and* The Good Granny Guide *by Jane Fearnley–Whittingstall, published by Short Books.*

FOUR

❧

how to

work and

have

a life

Having It All

We all hear of supermoms, those celestial beings who rise effortlessly up the career ladder, whose children are immaculately raised and whose marriages appear to be perfect. I just never get to meet them. For most of us, the most stressful time of our lives (but also—*never forget*—one of the most wonderful and rewarding, too) is the arrival of a first child. Even for the few who are well off enough to give up work and attend to their child full-time, it involves huge changes from their previous carefree, childless life. I shall never forget the utter loneliness that I felt after my first child was born and my husband used to kiss me goodbye as he set off for work, saying, "Bye—see you later." As the front door shut I knew I was going to be mostly alone with a small, demanding, crying, hungry baby for the next nine hours. I loved her more than I'd ever thought possible, but I hadn't anticipated the sense of isolation that being left alone with a small baby brings. After the companionship of a busy office, the lunches with girlfriends, the interesting work, the freedom to scurry to the theater, the exhilarating evening meetings (my husband was then much involved in politics), it was a huge shock. I was lucky in one sense in that I needed to work (at the time I didn't have the option of staying at home), so we got a nanny. I went back to my busy job and reclaimed much of my previous life, though I still feel guilty about not having been at home during the day for my children during those early years.

Since then, life for most women has become more difficult, not less. Few families can buy houses, or enjoy the sort of vacations and lifestyle that modern families aspire to, on just one average salary, so far more women are having to work. Also there are many more single parents having to bring up children alone. The statistics tell us that in 2006, some 14 million single parents in the United States were looking after 21.6 million children. For most of them going to work is usually not a luxury or a nice little cherry on the family cake, it's a necessity. Added to which, work is usually much, much more demanding than it used to be. All during my children's growing-up years I worked on Sunday newspapers or the weekend section of the *Financial Times,* which meant that I could almost always be home for bath, bed, and stories and, later on, for family dinners and talk of school, homework, practice, and so forth. These days most people I know work intolerably long hours— which is a huge problem whether they have children or not. British workers work the longest hours in Europe and a recent Amicus survey found that the effects on family life of long working hours, coupled with appalling commuting times, meant that most of those surveyed were too tired to enjoy their home, their families, their friends, or their hobbies.

Before this begins to sound depressing, I should also like to point out that one of the reasons that this situation has become such a problem is that the opportunities out there for women are so much greater. Life is richer and more complex, but the corollary is that it's often more stressful.

So what to do? The first thing is to accept that there are no magic bullets. You can't have it all. I truly don't think it is possible to have a glittering career (if it involves very long hours and lots of traveling), well-adjusted, happy children *and* a loving marriage or relationship, but I do think it's possible to have a medium career (that is, something that you can do in predictable hours without too much traveling) as well as happy, well-adjusted children and a good marriage. Since something's got to give, it seems to me that it's usually best for the family as a whole if the woman can bring herself to put her own career, even for a short time, on the back burner. Tough, I know, but I think that's the reality. Some women with fabulous careers ask their husbands to give up their own career to look after the children. This sometimes works, but does an alpha woman (or any woman, come to that) really want a meek, docile, beta house husband? I don't think so. It upsets the balance of power in the relationship in ways that don't psychologically suit either man or woman, in my view. And usually—but by no means always—it's in the family's interests for the man's career to be given most attention, for even in today's more emancipated environment men *usually* still have a greater earning capacity and wider horizons.

The choices facing women are hardest for the group that knows that slowing down or taking time off, even for just a few years, may mean giving up forever the chance of making it—if not to the top, then probably to where they want to be. Now that women are having children later (but this, as I don't need to tell you, also comes with the downside that they risk missing out on having children at all), it's possible in some careers to get high enough up the ladder to be able to take a smallish career break without losing out on the promotion stakes. Really high flyers can even risk taking complete career breaks—a wonderful thing to do for those whose confidence and abilities are exceptional. I know of one very successful young woman with four youngish children who went off with them and her husband for a whole year to wander around the world, but she knew that she was so employable that she'd have a choice in terms of work when she got home. He ran his own businesses, so he was going to be fine, too.

Most of us aren't so gifted or sought after and so the choices are tough, though at least today (unlike in my own child-rearing days) companies are more lenient in granting maternity leave and are obliged to give you your job back if you want it.

As you can see, there are no magic solutions—I can only offer thoughts. I know that I regret enormously that I wasn't more involved in the day-to-day minutiae of my children's lives—picking them up each day from school, taking them to gym class or swimming class, etc.—but at first I couldn't afford to give up work. By the time I could, I'd got to like my job a lot and got paid enough to mean that I could afford good child care.

But even full-time mothers need some down time, some time to themselves. Nobody, I think, finds full-time child care and domestic work a totally satisfactory way to spend their days and it's perfectly normal to want some time for your own hobbies, interests and friendships. Try to arrange for a grandparent to help, say, twice a week to give you some free time or, if that's not possible, organize swaps with other mothers—so that you have their child one afternoon a week in exchange for their having yours on another afternoon. As the child gets older, preschool beckons, whole mornings begin to become free and the world opens up again.

What is happiness except the simple harmony
between man and the life he lives.
—ALBERT CAMUS

TIME TO TAKE STOCK

Maybe it's worth taking time to think more carefully about what you really want in life. Do you most want a high-powered job? Who was it who said, "Be careful what you ask for, as you may get it"? If that's what you want, then take good stock of what you may very probably lose out on: a very close relationship with your children and possibly even with your husband/lover/partner as well. And are you intent on working because you have a great gift or skill (as a lawyer, surgeon, writer, stained-glass window maker, potter, or gardener) or because you really need the money? If it's money, or you think it's money, think more deeply about that, too. It may well be that your income really is absolutely essential—it is for many women—but it may also be that you're suffering from what these days is called "affluenza" ("a painful, contagious, socially transmitted condition of overload, debt, anxiety, and waste resulting from the dogged pursuit of more"). It's worth asking yourself how much money you *really* do need. After all, childhood is gone in a flash. As comedienne Ruby Wax once put it: "How much money do you have to make before it doesn't matter that your child sues you when he's twenty-eight for being missing in action."

Among my younger friends I know of several couples that consist of two high-powered bankers or two hugely successful lawyers (you get the picture), each of them earning more than enough to keep them comfortably in their houses, skiing vacations, and private-school tuitions, yet they see scarcely anything of their children. One or other of them is often on a plane; both often work late; and the households are kept afloat by relays of nannies, cooks, chauffeurs, gardeners, and the like. Private schools see this all the time—children who are materially spoiled beyond imagining, for whom half-terms are spent flying first class to the world's glamour spots, but who are emotionally more deprived than many children from the third world.

Take a moment to think about the correlation between money and happiness. There comes a time when working harder and therefore earning more results in lesser rather than greater happiness. In a fascinating survey carried out recently by London University, the researchers tried to establish what connection—if any—there was between money and happiness. Some of the findings weren't too surprising. Yes, for the very poor, enough money could measurably buy happiness, in that the difference between being able to afford your rent, food, and other basics and not being able to afford them is such a crucial leap that it is literally the difference between continuous, serious angst and a sense of ease and peace. *But* once most of those basics were taken care of, all sorts of other things made more difference to the sense of well-being of the people questioned. Most important of all was good health (which, the researchers found, was the equivalent to a pay raise of some £304,000, or about $600,000 a year), followed by marriage (the equivalent to earning an extra £54,000, or $100,000 a year), while living with somebody was even better (worth an extra £82,500, or $165,000 a year), and just chatting to a neighbor on a regular basis gave a sense of satisfaction equal to a pay raise of £40,000 ($80,000) a year.

Happiness, as we all know, comes from a complex combination of things, but at the heart lies love, friendship, good relationships with family and friends, a degree of security, and meaningful work—preferably doing something that you're good at. One friend once said to me that his dream for his children was that they would find a means of earning a living that they so enjoyed doing that it didn't seem like work; it was what they wanted to do anyway. That is the dream. . . . Few of us achieve it but it is possible.

Maybe you would be happier working less hard and living more simply, having more energy and time to spend with children, husband, lover or partner, friends and family. Think about it carefully—assess what gives you satisfaction, what makes you feel good. You might be surprised at some of the answers.

It's also worth adding up what it costs you to work—because working isn't cheap. You need to pay for transportation, for different sorts of clothes; you tend to spend more on fast food, cleaning, laundry, and all the rest. Again, the cost of working may amaze you.

> *Spend twice as much time*
> *and half as much money.*
> —A HEADMASTER IN AN ADDRESS TO PARENTS.
> IT APPLIES, HE POINTED OUT, AS MUCH TO
> THE PLUMBER AS TO THE BANKER.

IT'S NOT ALL BAD NEWS

On the plus side for working mothers, I would put the fact that both my husband and I spent every nonworking minute (and we were lucky that both our jobs involved pretty ordinary working hours) with our children and we always saw it as a treat and a pleasure, never a burden—evenings, weekends, and vacations were sacrosanct—we were never looking for ways of "dumping them." We were also able to live rather more amply than we would have been able to do without my income.

Our children got to be self-reliant and independent when they were quite young. I remember one of my son's tennis coaches being stunned that a nine-year-old boy could cross the city on his own, turn up on time with the right clothes and rackets, and cheerfully set off home again on his own. It makes me blanch a bit to think about it now—but then it seemed quite normal.

I *think* our children like the fact that not just their father but also their mother has a life, an independence, an income of her own. I never had a day when I didn't worry about my own mother, and I really don't think mine worry about me at all— which I think is a nice gift to give them. When the children have left home, work is a big consolation. The money's nice but so is the sense of purpose, the companionship and the continually expanding horizons. So while I miss those years when the children were at home—the happiest of my life—I'm not totally bereft now that they've flown the nest. I have another life, *and* (something I much enjoy) another income, which buys them—and their children—some pretty nice treats.

GETTING HELP

Sleep Problems

For working women probably the most stressful time of their lives is when the moment comes after the birth of a baby to go back to work. Sleep—or lack of it—is an all-consuming obsession. Even new mothers not going back to work find that getting enough sleep dominates their lives.

Try to establish a routine. Getting a baby used to learning to go to sleep by himself or herself is an essential survival tactic—for you and him. Babies, unless they're ill, are tougher than one thinks. After about six months, if there are no digestive problems, a baby should be able to last the night without a feed or drink.

Never let a baby become accustomed to sleeping in your bed—you'll never have a good night's sleep and it will be a nightmare trying to persuade him back to his own bed.

Some children are better sleepers than others and some mothers are naturally better disciplinarians than others. If you have problems, try to get them sorted out early on—for your own sanity and the baby's. My own daughter, and several other people I know, have been driven to distraction by babies who didn't sleep, but there are children's sleep consultants who can

help. In Los Angeles, Jennifer Waldburger and Jill Spivack at
Sleepy Planet (310-573-9474 and at www.sleepyplanet.com),
offer personal advice, either in person or over the phone. Those
who have used Sleepy Planet say it's money well spent every time.

☞ *When you're truly desperate, it's worth knowing that Night Nannies, too,*
will come to your rescue—for a fee. They're a godsend if you can afford them.
They know just how to calm a fractious baby and soothe him or her into good
sleeping habits. Check out www.gentlehandschildcare.com
for a list of regional contact details.

Child Care

The biggest problem facing the working mother is child care.
All those years ago, I could afford a live-in nanny on a good income but it was certainly not that of a lawyer or a banker. That
has become much more difficult today—nannies cost a king's
ransom, with massive bribes (apartments of their own, pricey
cars, first-class flights, etc.) from the new breed of hugely afflu-
ent bankers making it harder for those on average salaries to
compete. All the evidence is that small babies need one-on-one
care. Those who are looked after by their own mothers, or a
dedicated nanny, granny, or caregiver, at least until the age of
one, thrive much better than those who have to compete for attention with other babies and toddlers in the average nursery.
This, I am afraid, is an inconvenient fact. Numerous other
studies have shown that lack of proper parental love and care in
the early years can affect children's performance and sense of
psychological well-being all their lives. So I worry about a
whole generation of babies being brought up in crèches, however well run. It may be that in the early years you need to
think of part-time work, if you can organize it or afford it, or
do some work from home. Employers are becoming more family friendly and some now offer flextime, while certain quite
high-powered jobs can sometimes be organized as a job share

between two women, giving each of them precious time at home with their children as well as the stimulus of work and the benefit of income.

There is no short and sweet answer to this problem. The options are few and come down to a full-time nanny (expensive, but if you find the right one, the most reassuring and flexible solution); grannies or other family members; caregivers or day nurseries; and day care. All present some risks and obviously the quality of the person you choose is key (are they reliable, kind, energetic, honorable; do they like children, etc.), so taking up references is absolutely crucial. Partly you have to go by gut instinct, partly by their credentials (nurseries and day-care providers are carefully regulated), and partly by personal references. I don't think a day nursery is suitable for a child under one who still needs close one-to-one care, but I know that some mothers have no option. As the child gets older and more sociable, day nurseries have lots going for them. However, the best ones fill up fast so the time to check them out is the minute you know you're pregnant.

Nevertheless, you will still have to resign yourself to the fact that you will always feel guilty. When you are at work, you'll be worrying about the children, and when you're at home, you'll be worrying about work. It comes with the territory and I know of no way around it.

The other problem, which looms up later and which new mothers often don't take into account, is that teenagers are more, not less, needy than small children. Just because they don't have to be watched every minute of the day doesn't mean they don't still very much need close relationships with their parents. After all, nobody else can be expected to be as sensitive or as caring about their well-being or as alert to any looming problems as you, their parents. They need time with their parents; they should have frequent chances to talk to them and bring up things that may be worrying them. An au pair or a nanny who, if good, can provide for the wants of a small child is much less able to be emotionally satisfying for a teenager. So try to organize ways of keeping in as close touch with your teenage children's interests and needs as you can.

> *It would be terribly sad, wouldn't it, to look back on your life in films and not know your children? For me there's nothing more . . . lovely or rewarding than seeing my children grow up . . . and they only grow up once, remember.*
> —AUDREY HEPBURN

THROWING MONEY AT THE PROBLEM

Here, of course, that old bugbear—money—is important. You can't throw money at the problem if you don't have enough of it. But *even* if you do have enough of it, I think there are only certain problems for which it is decent to use money to buy your way out of trouble. It is *not,* in my view, decent to pay other people to deal with a difficult child who is probably just longing for more attention from his or her parents. It is *not,* in my view, decent to pay other people to go to sports games, read bedtime stories, take him to the all-important school interview or generally do the things that are crucial to a child's sense of being loved and valued by her parents.

But if you have the sort of job that takes all the hours that God gives and you earn enough, then for heaven's sake buy the services of the cleaner, the gardener, or the cook, so that those chores are taken care of, leaving you with as much time as you can muster for the people who should, after all, be what matter most in life—your nearest and dearest, whether wife, husband, children, siblings, or mother and father.

If you need to and can run to it, it may be worth spending a one-time sum to get the house properly sorted—unless you're one of those naturally organized people whose closets are immaculate and whose files are in tip-top order (see chapter 5). A declutter expert or even a life coach could show you not only where you've gone wrong but how to get your priorities right.

If you can afford it, some of the concierge services that now abound (www.quintessentially.com to name but one) will organize things like sending presents, booking air fares and vacations, plan house moving, and anything else that can be delegated. Consider It Done (888-860-3663 and at www.consider itdone.com) will provide support services at home. They'll take over household chores, organize garden maintenance, or get house sitters in when you're away, as well as provide secretarial services at home.

Merry Maids (www.merrymaids.com) will give the house a good clean, taking in everything from light bulbs to dusty corners.

Remember the maxim of Mr. Micawber, in Charles Dickens's *David Copperfield:*

"Annual income twenty pounds, annual expenditure nineteen nineteen six, result happiness. Annual income twenty pounds, annual expenditure twenty pounds ought and six, result misery."

Keeping control of one's spending is one of the most obvious ways of reducing stress.

GET ORGANIZED

Most of us can't afford to pay other people to do these things and so we have to do them ourselves. Making lists helps enormously. The busier your life, the more you need lists. There's something so satisfying about ticking items off. One very successful man I know says he tackles his list by starting off, when he's fresh and the day is young, with the things that he least wants to do. The day, then, can only get better and better.

Planning ahead also helps. Get the shopping sorted by organizing a weekly list with Peapod (www.peapod.com) or Safeway (www.safeway.com). It's a bore the first time around but once it's all set up it saves you hours and, best of all, you don't have to worry about parking or hauling all the heavy stuff home.

When I ran what I call an "establishment" (two children, a nanny, the cleaner, my husband, and me), I used to plan food quite carefully at the weekends. As I cooked, say, Sunday lunch, I'd be cooking something else for the week ahead—a soup, a casserole, a lasagna, and what in Britain we call pudding (and which my American editor has indulged me and allowed me to call it here and throughout the book, even though you know it as "dessert")—so that at least the first two or three days didn't need much thinking about. If I had the occasional easy weekend, I'd stock up the freezer by making, say, two batches of casserole, one for the meal that day, the other for the freezer. A freezer—a big new excitement then—was a fantastic asset. If properly stocked, it meant that you never ran out of bread, butter, or most of the basics. These days fast food has gotten so much better that you scarcely need to cook if you don't feel like it—*but* it is infinitely more expensive than cooking from scratch.

Having a tidy house saves many crucial minutes a day (as Dawna Walter, the closet guru, once put it, "If you can find what you need exactly when you need it you'll save hours a week"). By "tidy," I don't mean the sort of anal house where nothing is ever out of place, but a basic tidiness, with closets reasonably sorted, so that you can find sheets or washcloths when you need them, where files are in order and clothes hung up.

Tidiness can be made easier by developing a habit of tidying as you go along so that you don't let the mess develop from a minor nuisance into a major one, which means clearing a mini minefield every week, as one woman I know used to do (she let everything build up until Saturdays, which were an absolute nightmare of dirty dishes, piles of laundry, stuff all over the floor and so forth). That sort of major clearing-up effort involves big chunks of time and is seriously dispiriting.

I, for instance, try to do little bits of tidying when I have a few spare minutes. While I wait for a kettle to boil I might, say, tidy a kitchen drawer or do the dishes waiting in the sink. Putting things away after you've used them is one of the simplest ways of keeping disorder at bay. Above all, you don't want to have the sort of house that gets so untidy that you dread the unexpected visitor or that is so cluttered that you can't find the kettle because it's covered in junk.

Learn to Compromise

We've already seen that having it all isn't an option. There aren't enough hours in the day, so it's essential to learn to compromise. This means working out what really matters—whether time with your child, your work, a perfect home, seeing your friends, couple time, or hobbies. The balance between all these things will need to be rethought once you have children. If your work isn't all that rewarding, why not take the chance (*if* you can afford to) to take a year or so off to look after your child or children while you regroup your energies and rethink your career plans. You may have to see slightly less of your friends, go less often to the theater, give up time in the gym and stop worrying about your house looking so perfect. Remember, childhood goes in a flash.

If you're a working mother, on an average income, you can't run your house as if there were a battalion of servants or as if you were at home all day. So don't try. Children would much rather you had fun with them, read to them, taught them to ride a bike, or took them hiking, than that the house was a shrine to cleanliness. Nobody ever lay on their deathbed wishing they'd spent more time cleaning, whereas plenty die regretting that they didn't spend more time with the people they loved. If you're short of time, work out ways of making the provision of meals less bothersome. Children don't need elaborate food. They need fresh, healthy food that doesn't have to be labor intensive—simple roasts, pastas, grilled fish, and fresh vegetables can all be turned out without too much effort if you plan ahead. Children don't have to have two hot meals a day—cold food is just as nourishing as hot. Nobody dies if the clothes aren't ironed—buy as many noniron clothes for the children as possible so that they can just be tossed in the machine, dried and put back on. If you can afford it, use dry-cleaning and laundry services that deliver (www.pressed4time.com and www.1-800-dryclean.com).

You may have to settle on giving up for a few years some things that you care about. I seem to remember that for a long period we were never able to go on a proper walk (small children walk too slowly) or play tennis (because it would have meant leaving them on the weekend when we wanted to be with them) and I almost never had time to read a book, but the years flashed by and soon we were into doing most things with the children (tennis, skiing, hiking, playing chess and card games, and the like). The time really does go quickly, so give up some of your treats for a few critical years for the greater pleasure of spending time with your children. Remind yourself every so often how fast childhood goes and how much time (if you're lucky) you will have to yourselves after the children have left.

It's not having what you want,
it's wanting what you've got.
—SHERYL CROW

STRESS RELIEVERS

Exercise: It's the best reliever of stress there is and besides, it makes one feel much more able to cope with stress than slobbing around on a sofa ever does. The secret is to find something you like (such as swimming, yoga, tennis, golf, or hiking) and, if all else fails, book yourself a personal trainer. It's expensive and possibly self-indulgent, but if it's the only thing that gets you moving, it's essential.

Hobbies: It helps to have a passion, something you love to do that isn't connected to work. I know it's hard to justify the time if you're already trying to juggle work and family life, but perhaps it's worth each partner thinking about giving the other a present of something like two hours a week when they can do whatever they like: joining a book club, going to the theater, or having a piano, painting, or photography lesson.

Massage: It's not cheap, but if you can afford it there are few better ways (other than exercise!) to soothe the nerves. Quite apart from its more serious benefits (helping with stiffness, knotted areas in the neck or back, "bad" knees, etc.), it gives you an hour or an hour and a half when you have nothing to do but relax. It's been known for thousands of years that touch can be a powerful healer. For the elderly in particular, who live alone and have lost those closest to them, and so no longer have any physical relationships in their life, the touch of a masseur's hand can help to reduce depression, enhance the immune system, and ease pain.

Spa treatments: Apart from massage, as far as I'm concerned most other spa treatments are entirely frivolous, which isn't to say that some people don't enjoy them hugely. If they're what makes you feel better and you can afford them, why not indulge from time to time but remember that you can get much the same benefit at home for a fraction of the price. Book in some "me" time, lock the bathroom door, light some candles, turn on the radio, or the iPod or whatever gives you pleasure, and soak in a sea of Ren's Moroccan Rose Otto bath oil (available from www.annemichele.com) for as long as you feel like it.

FIVE

home, sweet home

What Is a Home?

To me, having grown up in a fractured family as more or less a nomad in South Africa, without a secure family home as a refuge, my own home is now everything. It's so much more, though, than four square walls and so much more than mere possessions. It's a sanctuary for me and the people I care about. It's where I feel safe, where I'd rather spend my time than in any six-star glossy hotel. It's where I like to think my family and friends can find tranquility, warmth and laughter, where I love to share food and wine and stories. As the outside world becomes more complex, most of us increasingly need the enveloping comfort of home. The current spate of what one commentator called "decorexia" (an obsession with the house and its contents) is, I think, symptomatic of more than just another field for competitive consumer spending; it is also an indication of our need for our own safe world. We're looking for ways to order our living spaces in ways that suit our particular lives, our families, our needs, our desires.

But a home is not a static place. It is the canvas on which we paint our personalities. As we all travel more, this influences the way we live and adds another layer to the things we surround ourselves with. In this way we change and grow, and our home evolves. For a home is also the storehouse of our family histories, a living archive that holds the treasures of our personal lives. Every picture, every book, every object tells a story. It speaks of where we've been and who we are, of what we mean to each other and of how we relate to the world around us.

I love best the sort of houses that are particular and truthful—and by that I mean that they're honest expressions of who the owners are. They've filled it with things they love and that have meaning. They haven't chosen the armoire, the painting, or the chaise longue solely to impress or created an environment that isn't an entirely truthful representation of who they are. The houses I like lack pretension, and they have no status symbols for the sake of them. That doesn't mean to say that some of them don't have some stunning and expensive pieces, but they're there because the owners truly love them, have perhaps discovered the designer/maker themselves, have brought them home in high excitement after some long journey and not merely plonked them down because they're a trendy thing to own.

> *I have no recipe for how to combine things. But you must be sincere. And if you are, strangely, it will succeed.*
>
> —ANDRÉE PUTMAN,
> THE EXCEEDINGLY ELEGANT FRENCH DESIGNER

Practical observation tells me that Andrée Putman (above) is absolutely right. Choose things you really, honestly love and somehow they'll work together. Our own house is filled with a very eclectic collection of things: a five-hundred-year-old stone gentleman from Bali, a very recent Edmund de Waal ceramic installation given to me by my children, African masks and tribal stools, a Victorian wrought-iron child's cot upholstered and turned into a small sofa, an antique French bedstead, pictures that range from the first (frankly rather strange) print I ever bought for just $25 to one or two rather lovely drawings and paintings inherited from my father. Strangely, they seem to work together.

As you can tell, I care about our home. The present one isn't where our children were born or were mostly brought up, but when we bought it they were still—just—at home and they set out from here, at an interval of three years apart, to Cambridge and the bigger, wider world, coming back often enough to make us feel that their lives and presences are part of the history of the house.

When it comes to style my tastes are relatively simple, veering towards the boho and the romantic. I admire austere simplicity when it's beautifully done, but can't quite bring it off myself. Nor do I like anything too grand or too imposing. I do mind tremendously—too much, my husband would say—about how things look. I absolutely empathize (again) with Andrée Putman when she says, "Of course, I love seven pillows behind me, but physical comfort is never the first thing. I prefer spiritual comfort, by which I mean space, light (natural, as well as artificial), contrast of textures, and pure lines. I never look for literal comfort, but for something that allows my mind to rest." I know just how she feels. I'm irked to an irrational degree by things that don't look right and not nearly enough by things that don't work quite so well.

I think I'm pretty good at getting things to look interesting but I am, I confess, not so good at organizing the practicalities. In an ideal world I'd have them both. I'd love to have loads of storage, enough working space in the kitchen, a small table and a light wherever one is needed, really comfy chairs and sofas, and all the other practical and technical things that these days make such a difference. On the other hand, perfection is often a little dull. (Remember what Truman Capote said about Babe Paley: "Babe Paley had only one fault: she was perfect; otherwise she was perfect.") There's something about a house being an ongoing project that is rather beguiling. If it were all done in one fell swoop a certain something, I can't help feeling, would be removed from daily life. I can't imagine buying one of those "turnkey" apartments where you just hand over a check and everything is done for you. Where's the fun in that?

In any event, getting it right is complicated, requiring an immense amount of planning, not to mention an address book more than a foot thick. But all the best and most interesting houses evolve over time. We married very young with no money and such cash as there was went to the children and childcare, so for years we had very little furniture and could afford few luxuries. But over the decades we have accumulated things—presents that we've given each other and that our children and others have given us; pictures we've inherited; odds and ends I've brought back from my journalistic wanderings—and all these objects, I like to think, make our house particular and personal. So don't be impatient. The best houses take time. If they're to be true expressions of who you are, then it can't be done overnight. Build it up, layer upon layer, as your life evolves.

Here I try to pass on just some of the lessons I've learned as I've grappled with trying to keep our much-loved house looking good and working well.

Fundamentals

The thing I always remember about my mother, who never had much money but who always looked a dream (she never weighed more than a hundred pounds from the day I was born), was that she made the small and not very prepossessing apartments she lived in seem warm and welcoming because she always filled them with books and music, flowers, fruit, and chocolates. (Nowadays I'd add wine, but in those innocent days I hadn't discovered its pleasures, and neither had she.) None of those are really expensive (particularly in South Africa) and I've always thought that in some ways you don't need a lot more than that. They are all things that we require for mental nourishment, for sensuous comfort and for aesthetic pleasure. If you've got those, you're in clover. But there are other things that make a difference: warmth (how I remember, in the days before ubiquitous central heating, the frozen rooms that greeted me when I first landed in the U.K.), candles, plump cushions, comfy beds, fine sheets, good soap, great coffee, a great big kitchen table, and so on. In addition to those, a certain level of order and tidiness really helps (squalor isn't restful), while a few touches of glamour add the magic.

Generosity, whether of the mind or the purse (and in my experience they tend to go together), is hugely appealing, and so it is with houses. It shows. There is nothing more attractive than a warm and welcoming home—it's more important than worrying about whether the house is scruffy or down-at-the-heels. There's nothing more off-putting than the skimpy bowl of fruit, the mean-sized towels, the cheap soap, or the inadequate central heating. The converse is also obviously true: great piles of fluffy white towels in a bathroom, wonderful soap, and ample hot water are hugely comforting, while a house filled with the essentials—music, books, fruit, and flowers—is so inviting that you could (almost) forget the furnishings.

And remember: it's a home, not a museum. It's for living in, not for looking at. Have things you love.

Touches of Magic

It is my common observation that nothing spells death to an interior more than the small, the mean, and the dinky. A touch of grandeur does wonders for even the smallest of homes. Just as the classic technique for any fashion brand trying to reinvent itself is to dip into its archive, to take some classic designs and play about with scale, upsizing and downsizing, the same is true for the house. Playing about with scale (what one might call an *Alice in Wonderland* ploy) can add a touch of magic to almost any room.

For the marvelously sumptuous Turkish designer Alidad, getting the scale right is where good design starts. "If scale is not right, it can kill a room. When in doubt, overscale—it always works. I usually go to extremes. If a client has a small room and wants it to look special, I choose the biggest patterns I can find, and the large table or commode that will only just squeeze through the door. You can visually expand a room by cheating the eye; overscaling seems to push back the walls and ceilings." This also applies to big-patterned wallpaper and to accessories. A couple of D.C.-based designers, Robert Cole and Sophie Prevost, used "the grandest, tallest, definitely overscaled lounge chair in the tiniest drawing-room . . . and it looked wonderful. It actually made the room feel bigger."

Tables can be given a bit of added theatre by using oversized hurricane lamps as candle-holders—small and medium just look conventional, but once you go large the change in atmosphere is dramatic. Chunky glasses, big mirrors, oversized platters, and even huge fat poles for curtains with great big rings are all different ways of imbuing a house with a sense of generosity and making sure a room never looks bland.

Chandeliers—not grand, pompous ones that look as if they were devised for formal reception rooms in so-called grand hotels, but enchanting little antique ones from France or Italy—lend an enchantment to almost any room. Dining rooms and living rooms are obvious contenders for their charms, but some of the most sensuously welcoming bathrooms I know sport a chandelier in the middle. I have one over my own dining table and it gives me joy daily. The light is delicious (on the wall opposite we have a Venetian mirror and the light reflected back and forth is wonderful) and it is on a dimmer switch so we can have slightly mysterious half light when we need it. Oversized chandeliers can sometimes work. Philippe Starck put a black glass chandelier in a sugar-pink room at the Baccarat headquarters in Paris and it looked fabulous. And if chandeliers aren't right think about some scintillating art deco lights—the glittering chrome and glass remind one irresistibly of movies, the glamour of Hollywood, of Fred and Ginger in their heyday.

Huge mirrors leaned nonchalantly against a wall are currently a fashionable interior prop and very good they look too. A giant Buddha or a statue add grace and grandeur to a room. They don't need to be expensive. All across the country there are antique shops, or what the French call *brocantes,* offering old mirrors for not a lot of money. And speaking of France, the provincial antique fairs (except Ile-sur-la-Sorge, which is now almost as expensive as Fifth Avenue) that are held at intervals all through the summer are a great source of old mirrors, old linen and all sorts of enchanting odds and ends. In the United States many a designer and style aficionado (Donna Karan and Paul Smith to name but two) makes regular pilgrimages to the incredible flea market that is held in Pasadena's Rose Bowl on the first Sunday of every month (1570 East Colorado Boulevard, Pasadena, California).

If you can't find things large enough on their own to be eye-catching, grouping them in multiples, even if they're fairly common or garden objects, gives them a visual importance that often works. One African mask can look a bit silly but five look dramatic. The interior designer Kelly Hoppen once told me that sometimes she would buy huge glass vases from Habitat (or you could try Crate & Barrel) in threes or fives (somehow odd numbers work better than even), group them asymmetrically and they would look divine. I copied her, bought three huge glass vases for very little and filled them with giant fake deep red amaryllis (about $10 a stem), and put them on a landing table. They look, I think, terrific. At the Conran Shop, you might come across a dining table embellished with a vast array of different-sized glass candlesticks, none of them expensive, and the mass is what makes the magic. I was once in a room that was fairly austere—lots of white paint and bare floorboards— but the mantelpiece was lined with a row of Buddhas that looked interesting and exotic, and added a bit of panache. "Where," I enquired of the owner, "did they come from?" Marks & Spencer, she said, without a blush. (Marks & Spencer being, if you're not aware, a British institution, to whit, a reasonably priced high-street chain where famously everybody from duchesses to shop girls normally buy their knickers—and it all goes to show that these things can be found if you keep your eyes peeled in cheap places.)

In yet another all white and cream room with painted wooden floors, the whole room was saved from austerity and a certain bleakness by the addition of a single—but very beautiful—old, carved armoire. In a conventional room with conventional antiques the old armoire would have contributed no drama, but in its austere white setting it seemed theatrical and wonderful. In another equally clean-lined room one brilliant quirky piece, in this case a silvered curving chest of drawers, added the buzz that the room so badly needed.

Quite often a room can be enlivened by changing the eye level. If all the furniture is of a similar height the effect is dull and monotonous, so lead the eye upwards (particularly in a high-ceilinged room or one where there is a particularly beautiful cornice or ceiling) by choosing a tall piece of furniture or erecting something like a high screen. And never forget candles, about which more later (page 245). Even the dullest interior can be turned, at night, into a wonderland if there are enough candles to shed their wonderfully soft, flickering light. You can buy lots of small cheap glasses (more contemporary than silver candelabra) or, slightly more expensively, lots of glass candlesticks and the light from the candles will be reflected off the glass in a magical way. Instead of small Georgian candlesticks, go for less conventional, quirkier ethnic ones—oversized, of course.

If you have space—on a landing, in a corner—think about doing something that I once saw in Biki Oberoi's Udaivilas Hotel in Udaipur, which is to have a table given over entirely, come the evening, to a massed array of lighted candles of various shapes and sizes. Its sole purpose was to create an air of magic.

The important thing is for a room to have visual variety so it doesn't do to use only large pieces, the point being that you want contrast rather than uniformity. Symmetry and asymmetry also need to be balanced, because too much of either is simply dull. In very large rooms try splendid architectural pieces—carved wooden doors, pillars, huge urns, big fireplaces, even complete staircases. They can often be found at the suppliers of architectural salvage (try Olde Good Things—their main warehouse is in Scranton, Pennsylvania, but they have locations in New York, Los Angeles, and Miami; 888-233-9678). Everything it sells has the immense advantage of being one-of-a-kind, and so is to be doubly treasured.

☞ *If you can't afford serious art, blow up and hang on one hall a favorite black and white photograph or picture, megasize—it'll look dramatic and twice as important. There are now plenty of companies that will do it for you (see chapter 7, "Perfect Presents").*

Ilse Crawford, the designer behind Babington House in Somerset in the U.K. and Soho House in the Meatpacking District in New York, seems effortlessly to conjure up magic. She combines a sense of cool with an updated version of old-world glamour. In her very white rooms in Soho House there are zebra skins on the floors (there is something very sensual about animal skins; I suppose it was Elinor Glyn and her tiger skin rug that did it), lots of mirrored surfaces, and the odd piece of baroque or quirky furniture. (If you don't fancy a zebra skin on the floor, even though the skins should come only from zebras that have died a natural death, consider a cowhide.)

Texture is another way of providing a sense of luxe, which is partly what glamour is about. Cushions are possibly the least expensive way to inject some instant allure. Many retail stores—Bloomingdale's, Pottery Barn, and Restoration Hardware—often have wonderfully rich cushions, silk quilts, and bedspreads at fantastic prices. Have a look at www.comfort house.com.

And finally, flowers, flowers, flowers.

Economy Glamour

Suzanne Imre, editor of a leading British interior design magazine, *Livingetc,* offers ten ways to add a touch of magic without breaking the bank.

1. Stain floorboards in the darkest wood stain you can possibly find (I use Dulux Trade Ebony stain) and paint walls and skirting boards in a fresh, pure white (Farrow & Ball's All White).

2. Fit elegant, smoked-glass doorknobs on all internal doors. Buy the most expensive ones you can afford as they will still be cheaper than changing all the doors!

3. Hang a large, mirrored disco ball in the hall (Jade Jagger has one in her house in Ibiza, while John Hiscox, a leading British property developer, has one overhanging his swimming pool) to create a little sparkle and tongue-in-cheek amusement each time you walk into your home. (Get them from www.stagelightingsource.com.)

4. Glam up your kitchen with nothing more than elbow grease: polish all your stainless steel to a high shine, from plug sockets to cooking utensils. They will reflect the light and help make the room look instantly smarter.

5. Have fun with scale and never go for the middle road. Opt for the size that will create dramatic impact in a particular space: mini mosaics or huge slabs of stone in a bathroom; a narrow delicate armchair or an oversized, squashy sofa for a sitting room; or try the juxtaposition of a grand, wide chandelier in a long, slim hallway.

6. Plain white sheers at windows always look effortlessly elegant. Hang them high above the window frame and let them cascade down to tumble on the floor, creating a long slim shape that makes the ceilings appear higher too.

7. A beautifully scented home is the ultimate flirtation with the senses. After dark, dim the lights (never use anything brighter than 60 watts), and light scented candles in hallways, sitting rooms, and bathrooms.

8. Give a tired, but interestingly shaped, piece of wooden furniture a touch of Italian gloss by lacquering or car-paint spraying it in brilliant white, sexy black, or deep ruby red. Find a local car mechanic who can help.

9. White kitchens are simply the best when it comes to modern interiors, but they can run the risk of looking sterile at times. Break up a plain space and add a shot of style in the form of a mirrored mosaic backsplash. It guarantees instant edge.

10. Buy a number of inexpensive black picture frames in differing sizes and mount your favorite black and white photos in them. Group the frames artfully on the wall or, for a more casual look, lean them on shelves, overlapping if you like.

MIX AND MATCH

There's something very staid and old-fashioned about having everything that matches. Think of the traditional dining table, sideboard, and chairs all perfectly matched—very, very boring, very last century. Mix a traditional table with funky chairs—Philippe Starck's Ghost chair, or even his Mademoiselle chair (both done for Kartell), or the Tulip chairs that Eero Saarinen designed all those years ago for Knoll. You can even mix the chairs themselves, providing they're all in roughly the same mood. If you have a table the right size but it looks staid and down-at-heel (in an unattractive way, not a divine shabby-chic kind of way), you can get it sprayed in a brightly colored lacquer—even deep shiny black.

At the Milan Furniture Fair a few years ago, all the trendiest tables had red lacquered legs; they looked great (still do) so you could update a dull table by just spraying the legs. I saw a wonderful table the other day that had clearly once had a shabby pine top but it had been overlaid with a beaten metal top and a whole gaggle of design journalists were looking at it agog. We all loved it. It had so much more personality than something too new and shiny from a snazzy showroom. And, of course, with dining tables size and proportion are more important than looks because you can always cover the top with a gorgeous cloth.

The three-piece suite has long ago died a death, but it reminds us that a varied collection of sofas and chairs is infinitely more interesting than matching sets. It needs a good eye, though, because while one, say, Louis XV chair in a very modern room looks brilliant, there are some styles that just don't mix. Usually if a piece is attractive enough in itself, it will blend with other things of equal quality. It's good, too, to put the odd antique in with the resolutely modern—or vice versa. It livens the interior up no end.

China and tableware, too, are much more fun if they're mixed up together instead of that "wedding-present," matching-set look. I first saw the charm of this more boho approach to dining tables some years ago in one of those quintessentially shabby-chic English country houses where the table was laid with a disparate collection of antique plates, silver and glass. I presumed that over the years some pieces had been broken and others had gone missing, but as it was the sort of house where there would have been plenty of different sets, I now think the owners simply put together whatever seemed to look good on the day. It looked wonderful.

Shortly after that I began to collect vintage blue and white plates from the old pottery companies whenever I came across them. Each and every one is different. I went on collecting over the years from various antique fairs and stalls, and I bring them out when I'm not in resolutely modern mode and want a table that looks not so much chic as pretty and inviting. Wedgwood has a very modern, avant-garde take on the harlequin notion with its selection of plates, each sporting a different portion of a traditional Wedgwood pattern, yet all working together because they come in the same color range. While it's fun to mix your own sets, try to keep the mood fairly similar. If you want to collect old china, it's worth looking at www.replacements .com.

And then there are glasses. In our house we're big fans of Riedel's austerely elegant wine glasses (each shape is beautifully tailored to enhance the grape type, so there is one glass for, say, Bordeaux, another for white burgundies and so on) and we always restock during the Harrod's sale when they are about half price. I also have a collection of wonderfully ornate seconds made in Florence that didn't cost very much. They're all in varying shades of green with rich baroque twirls of gold and come in different shapes and sizes. I don't bring them out when we're serving very fine wines (in which case, in my view, only Riedel will do), but I love them just the same. If you ever go to Venice or Florence don't miss a chance to get some wonderful glass there, but if you don't think you'll be in Florence any time

216 Things I Wish My Mother Had Told Me

Quick Ways to Update Your Home

1. Change your china. This doesn't cost a fortune and can immediately change the look. Throw out (or better still store) the plain white (just a little boring now). Bring in color and modern shapes, and mix with antiques.

2. You can't afford to throw everything out but a few brilliantly chosen quirky accessories can update the look—a floppy resin vase-cum-sculpture by Gaetano Pesce, some extraordinary glass by somebody like by Massimo Micheluzzi, or a huge elliptical vase from Lino Sabattini. Think of it as adding Jimmy Choo shoes to an H & M dress.

3. Change the cushions. Get them beaded, embroidered, covered in buttons or pleats in colors that give the room a new look.

4. Change the look at the window. If you have blinds, consider adding some floaty sheers as well. If you have thick lined curtains, swap them for something lighter and fresher.

5. Art is what the Wall Street set seem to spend their money on. So can you. You don't have to buy the big names in the posh galleries. Scour the annual student shows at art colleges and buy before Larry Gagosian gets there, or go to Frieze Art and the other user-friendly art markets that are burgeoning everywhere. Blow up a large photograph or get www.imagekind.com (888-264-1446) or www.photowow.com (800-453-9333) to give you a blown-up version of an image of your choice to fill a whole wall. If you're a techno whiz, you can play about the computer to create, say, Andy Warhol—like images of your own and enlarge them.

(continues)

Quick Ways to Update Your Home (*continued*)

6. Change the floor. Pull up a fitted carpet and sand and paint the floorboards, or swap a dowdy rug for something more modern.

7. Changing the walls isn't expensive—you can slap wallpaper (currently very much back in vogue) over existing paint or repaint over paint. A vibrant paper on one wall is very "now."

8. Refresh the lighting. Throw out anything dowdy. It's amazing what one wonderful light can do—a charming chandelier, say, or Ferruccio Laviani's Bourgie lamp, or an old photographer's or dentist's light from an antique market.

9. You can refresh the look of a chair or sofa with a throw or blanket—using, say, an all-white bedcover on a sofa if you're tired of its existing color.

soon you could collect a disparate group of glasses every time you see ones you love in an antique store or market—in time you'll have a great collection.

Water glasses of different colors but the same style often look very pretty on a table and I've seen tables laid with a varied collection of antique silver all collected from antique fairs at different times. Shops such as Pier 1 (800-245-4595 for a catalog and at www.pier1.com) and Anthropologie (www.anthropologie.com) have collections of glasses that come in all different colors. Lekker (1317 Washington Street, Boston 02118; 617-542-6464; www.lekkerhome.com) sells bar glasses with rounded bottoms in packs of four, each a different color ($31).

The same principle applies to cutlery. While we were lucky enough to inherit a collection of some properly matching pieces, I still can't resist buying up small bits of silver, particularly Georgian, whenever I come across them at fairs or pass a likely looking antique shop. Buying cutlery in small doses means you don't have to fork out a vast sum all at once and gradually it mounts up.

TARA BERNERD'S GUIDE TO RENOVATION

Tara Bernerd is a sassy and clever designer, and her company, Target Living, www.targetliving.com, has carried out a large number of architectural and design projects—some for private homes, some for large corporations such as the Blackstone Company.

1. The Brief Stop, look, and think about the space. The most common mistake is to launch into choosing colors and new fabrics before you've worked out how to make best use of the space. Think about how you will use the room, all the functions it will need to fulfill (eating, sitting, watching television, entertaining, whatever). It seems obvious, but if you do this it will clarify your mind and the steps you need to take. Collect images of inspirational rooms from magazines to try to identify what pleases you.

2. The Layout Draw a scaled plan of the room. This is essential if you are considering renovating but it also enables you to try out, with scale models of the furniture, how best to furnish the room. For instance, if you were redesigning your living room, you might start off thinking of a sofa and armchairs, yet through drawing up different options you might find that an L-shaped sofa and larger character chair would work better. It should also help you plan a lighting and electrical layout.

3. The Specification With the plan in hand and an idea of your furniture layout, you need to consider flooring, wall treatment, hardware (door handles, etc). You should do this before you choose the final colors and fabrics.

Think of it as building up an artist's palette. If going for a wooden floor, for instance, consider the type and color impact that this will have on your choice of wall covering and so on.

4. Feature Treatment You might identify an area that you'd like to emphasize or make stand out in some way—perhaps a wall with a fireplace or a large back wall on which you might put a different color (paint or lacquer), wallpaper or even leather to make a feature of it. This is usually easiest on one wall, on columns, or an obvious stand-alone area.

5. The Fabrics With a layout and specification in mind you can start hunting for fabrics or leathers, the materials for the room, again building up your palette. Choose approximately three fabrics, making sure they are not all too busy. Usually one should be more detailed and the other two less patterned, and occasionally one of these may be a strong bold color for a little edge. These fabrics will become the blinds, sofa and armchair material, and will usually be the main color in the room. Try to get large samples, as tiny swatches can be deceiving.

6. Furniture With a plan of your furniture layout, this will help focus you as well as ensuring that what you buy fits. Be wary of the spontaneous purchase that often turns out to be a real problem, either by not fitting or simply being the wrong color. So look around, buy magazines and perhaps have a style in mind. Draw up a clear list of what you need as well as measurements.

It is helpful to have a small zipped bag with all your samples together so that you can check that things fit in with your scheme.

7. General Planning Design is a logical process so consider all the various timing implications, i.e., lead times and installation time. Some companies have maddeningly long lead times.

8. Builders/Professionals Do consider professional help —it can save you expensive mistakes. Always ask to see the previous work of companies that you're considering.

9. Have Fun Once you're organized, with a layout, a spreadsheet of all your items and their corresponding prices and timings, you should try to enjoy the process and not be scared of change.

10. Accessories Finally look at cushions, throws, plants, etc. These final details can lift a whole room: a terrific pile of funky trunks, a fantastic throw or edgy cushions. But remember that just as the wrong hat can kill a wonderful outfit, so these details can be deadly if not chosen with care. Be honest, buy sincerely here and stay with the scheme.

Paint

Until I started updating our West London terraced house about six years ago, I hadn't realized quite how sophisticated the matter of choosing paint had become. It's joined the long list of totemic products that are said to speak volumes about their owners. Even so, with the mass of choice around, it isn't always easy to find what you want if you have something very specific in mind. For instance, I knew I wanted a dark, almost black, green for our front door and chose the darkest green I could find on the usual color charts. It wasn't dark enough. It irked me daily until a friend, with wonderful taste, to whom I bleated about my disappointment at not finding the right color, said, "Oh, the color you want is Shop Front Green." She was right. It's perfect. It made me realize how hugely important it is to get colors right. Because most of us choose paint colors so seldom, we don't get enough experience to know how the color on the chart will look in a big mass up on a wall or in combination with other colors. I can't begin to mention every brand around but I list below the pros and cons of some of the companies I've used.

Farrow & Ball, 8475 Melrose Avenue, Los Angeles 90069; 323-655-4499; www.farrow-ball.com. The first company to lift paint into the realm of a status symbol, it is most famous for producing the first historic range of paints and for the much-admired depth and flatness of the finishes (achieved by making paints the old, traditional way with no vinyl or plastics). Farrow & Ball recommend buying sample pots to experiment with before you decide, for colors appear to change, according to the area of the surface and any other colors near by. If you have grand, or even just pretty, cornicing, it's worth thinking of painting it just with distemper. This gives it a wonderfully powdery finish, highlights the carving and, because it can be easily washed off, you don't get that build-up of paint that flattens the detailing. There's a complete range of floor paints, too, not to mention exterior paints.

Marston & Langinger, 117 Mercer Street, New York 10012; 212-965-0434; www.marston-and-langinger.com. Brilliant outdoor paints—masses of shades of greens, for instance, to choose from, from palest lettuce to darkest forest—for conservatories, sheds, or fences.

The Paint & Paper Library, Stark Wallcovering, D&D Building, 979 Third Avenue, New York 10022; 212-752-9000. Its Architectural Range is fantastic, and now I nearly always use paints from its range. It has done much of the hard work by grouping paints in coordinated ranges. It has also taken some of the classic neutrals and off-whites, with names such as Wattle, Ivory, Slate, Stone, Lead, Sand, and Clay, and produced each of them in four different shades. Interior designer Ann Boyd, for instance, who was once the taste behind Ralph Lauren interiors and is as sophisticated a designer as you could hope to find, almost always chooses paints for her clients from the Paint & Paper Library. "If you're trying to do different tones in the same room he makes it dead easy. I just use, say, Wattle 1, 2, 3, and 4 in different places." Most people use Shade 1 on the ceiling, 2 on the cornices, 3 on the walls, and 4 on the woodwork but some will put 3 on the cornice and 2 on the woodwork. Whatever you do, you'll know that they're all in the same family of tones.

Portola's Paints & Glazes, 12442 Moorpark Street, Studio City, California 91604; 818-623-9053; www.portolapaints .com. Lime washes and glazes are just the thing if you fancy the look of a faded Italianate villa. They are the most traditional paints of all, made the way paint was made before the intro- duction of plastics, so when they dry they have that soft, vel- vety look that you see on the walls of grand palazzos. Their line includes sixty colors but they'll also custom-mix a color to any specification.

Mass-market Versus Niche Paints

When a gallon of Sherwin Williams paint can be bought for under $35, you might wonder how it is that some people are prepared to pay more than twice the price for something that doesn't seem to have a lot more to recommend it than a fancier, more obscure name.

The key is to know when and where to use these paints. Many interior decorators—particularly those who work on large developments where price becomes a key issue—are skilled at picking the sophisticated colors from lines by compa- nies such as Sherwin Williams and Benjamin Moore.

The big brands have realized that it wasn't enough to swamp the market with choice—what the public wanted was more advice, more closely edited ranges. Which is why Dulux and Benjamin Moore, for instance, have a selection of designers and consultants who can give advice on everything from colors to fashion trends. Ilse Crawford, who as we've already seen is the taste behind the new Soho House in New York's Meatpacking District, is one of Dulux's consultants. She helps put together not only advice on trends but more importantly color stories (such as Jungle Engineering, which homes in on a very fashionable group of grayish/greenish colors) that make it easy for the customer to choose shades that work together. One of the problems of the huge ranges is that the choices are almost too great. "If you have plenty of time," says Ilse Crawford, "you could probably nearly always find the colors you want, but it does take time and these days for many people time is money."

Joanna Wood, an interior designer whose clients have tastes ranging across a vast spectrum, says that she can often find neutral colors in the mass-market brands. When it comes to deep colors, such as reds ("It's so hard to find a red that isn't too coral or too purple in the more commercial ranges"), she opts for Farrow & Ball: "There is a greater intensity of color—the paint itself is thinner, so you need more layers, but there's more pigment in it." On the other hand, Tara Bernerd, who runs Target Living and has done interiors for private as well as commercial clients, turns to Farrow & Ball for a really deep, intense black, Black Railings.

When it comes to exterior paints, Joanna Wood thinks that it's hard to find in commercial ranges the more appealing colors made by the conservatory-building company Marston & Langinger. "Their colors are just perfect for the country, with a fantastic deep yellow as well as a green that is perfect against nature's own greens."

Commercial brands, which in reality have to please the mass market, have to take into account considerations such as durability, which has an impact on the formulations. The upside is that marks are more easily washed off and the paints last longer. The downside is that for many people the colors aren't chalky or subtle enough. The price you pay for the subtler colors from the niche companies, for the chalky effects, for the deeper pigments, is that they will be less easy to clean and that you'll have to repaint more often.

Objective Sources of Advice

One of the best is www.paintquality.com, which has useful advice on the different sorts of paints and how to use them. The Benjamin Moore Web site (www.benjaminmoore.com) offers lots of advice as well as a service to help you plan the color scheme for your room. Benjamin Moore will also mix up any color you like (if you take along an example of the color, they will match it exactly) so you can get as swanky a color as you like for a mass-market price.

WALLPAPER

If you haven't been asleep you'll know it's back big time. There are all sorts of niche manufacturers (of which the most famous is Timorous Beasties at www.timorousbeasties.com, which takes the classic toile de Jouy formula and subverts it by using gritty urban images instead of the charming rustic scenes traditionally used). New Orleans company, Flavor Paper (www.flavorleague.com) does gorgeous hand-screened custom-made papers, some vintage inspired, some utterly contemporary, and it offers a fantastic service as well—any of their designs can be printed in any of a wide range of colors. However the big three—Waverly (www.waverly.com), Cole & Son (www.cole-and-son.com, which had a lot of fun updating and recoloring its traditional flocked papers), and Schumacher (www.fschu macher.com)—have all smartened up their acts no end with an immensely rich array for us all to choose from.

For real glamour it's hard to beat **De Gournay** (www.de gournay.com), which takes traditional Chinese scenes and hand-paints them almost any color you'd like. For sheer glamour come the evening, a dining room decorated in one of its wonderful silver, black and gray hand-painted papers is hard to beat. In London it is run from 112 Old Church Street, London SW3 6EP (+44 20 7352 9988) or in the States from 143 West Twenty-ninth Street, Seventh floor, New York 10001 (212-564-9750 for an appointment).

Florence Broadhurst was a brilliant Australian designer of wallpapers who was murdered in mysterious, unresolved circumstances back in the late 1970s. Fortunately a couple of passionate admirers, Helen and David Lennie, have bought the archive and are now reissuing the wallpapers. They're brilliantly colored, flamboyantly decorative and so of the moment that it's amazing to learn they were all designed way back before the 1970s. Find them at John Rosselli & Associates, 979 Third Avenue, Suite 1800, New York 10022; 212-593-2060.

Designers Guild (head office), 3 Lasimer Place, London W10 6QT; +44 20 7893 7400. While she can do a sophisticated neutral as well as anybody else, it's probably for her heart-lifting collection of brilliant blues, stinging greens, and absolutely luscious pinks and reds that Tricia Guild is best known.

BEDROOMS AND BEDDING

I believe the reason that most of us get carried away by hotel bedrooms is twofold. First, unless we're very unlucky in the hotel we choose, the bedrooms are usually rather bigger than our own back home, and second, when we arrive we are greeted with a pristinely ordered space. There is no underwear hanging over the chair, no piles of old newspapers (which, I'm ashamed to say, are usually by my side of the bed); there is nothing gathering dust under the bed; the surfaces are clear, the linen clean, and the whole atmosphere, *even* when the decor is dire (it happens), is usually, at the very least, tranquil. That's the element that I think we should aim to reintroduce to our bedrooms back home. Clear the space. If possible (ah, me, a dream that, alas, the arrangements of my own dear *schloss* make impossible), make a dressing room where the clothes, the jewelry, the essential things we all need, can be stored.

A designer friend has a bedroom with a clever device to introduce orderliness: behind the bed itself, which is not against the wall but juts a little way into the room, is a very large screen and behind the screen is the area where clothes are kept, books stored and where all the paraphernalia that contributes to an unrestful atmosphere is hidden from the eye. It works a treat.

Hotels have shown us, too, just how much difference a really large bed can make, something like six feet wide being the minimum for a high-end hotel these days. It may be expensive to start with (and certainly the linen doesn't come cheap, either), but a large bed is an investment in marital happiness and good sleep that one realizes should—over a lifetime—pay for itself hands down. The Four Seasons hotel group, for instance, had so many requests from guests to buy the beds in which they'd enjoyed such happy nights that it now runs a small side-line making and selling beds. If you're interested, you should call the gift shop at your nearest Four Seasons Hotel (www.four seasons.com).

Biki Oberoi's sumptuous hotels in Rajasthan (Rajvilas, Udaivilas, and Vanyavilas) have wonderfully seductive bed-rooms. (Some of the decorative objects, most particularly the ornate "silver" candlesticks used at Rajvilas, are on sale by pop-ular demand and these days many other hotels have followed suit.) Those hotels illustrate the emotional appeal of the ample four-poster, the fluffed-up pillows, the television placed just so, and appropriate ethnic touches so that each hotel is anchored in a specific geographical place. But above and beyond all the decorative flourishes, it is the generous space allotted for clothes and bathing that makes the rooms such a joy to inhabit and if we can replicate that at home (not often a possibility, I know), what a difference it makes.

And absolutely key—the thing that even the very best ho-tels often fall down on—is good lighting. The number of times that one arrives in a so-called five-star luxury hotel and is un-able to read in bed far, far outweighs the number of times that one can actually read with pleasure. Think about that when you're planning the bedroom. These days, too, there are minia-ture lights that allow one partner to read while the other dozes off—important for those whose sleep patterns don't coincide.

Guest Rooms

I happen to feel very strongly about these, having had both wonderfully comfortable experiences in friends' houses and also some of the roughest nights ever where our dear hosts clearly hadn't the faintest idea of what it is like to sleep in their own spare room. I'm a bit neurotic about this since in my own family there circulates the tales of the aunt whose guest bed was so uncomfortable that it became a family legend—nobody ever went to stay with her twice.

So, first, sleep in the spare room yourself at least once. See what needs work. Is there good lighting—good enough to read by? Are the curtains (or blinds) thick enough to let guests sleep properly? Is it warm enough? Airy enough? And, most importantly of all, is the bed comfortable? If it isn't, change it (this is not easy, I know, but Bloomingdale's will take away your old one as they deliver the new one). An extra bit of luxury is a television set—nothing is so spoiling, in my view, as being able to watch the late-night news from one's very own bed. Put an extra blanket across the bed in case the guest needs it if the temperature drops. Have lots of delicious pillows—nothing looks so welcoming as huge square continental pillows encased in crisp white antique pillowcases. See below for more on bed linens. Don't palm guests off with easy-wash, no-iron polyester—give them really delicious pure cotton. You can buy it inexpensively from Macy's, Linens 'n' Things or Bed, Bath & Beyond. And make sure there is a wastepaper basket.

Little luxuries aren't expensive, either—a tin of cookies, a bowl of fruit, a fluffy white robe, slippers, a hot-water bottle, some really good books, a bottle of water, even (*quel luxe*) a little decanter of whisky.

☞ *If you can't run to enough spare rooms to cater for everybody who wants to come and stay (we now, for instance, have five small grandsons, which means that if they all come together we run out of beds), track down some foldaway beds, which you can bring out when needed. Other good solutions are those single beds with a drawer below that pulls out to become a second bed when it's needed.*

LINEN

And still she slept an azure-lidded sleep,
In blanched linen, smooth and lavender'd.

—JOHN KEATS, "THE EVE OF ST. AGNES"

I am of the opinion that one of life's little luxuries—one that a lot of us can afford—is freshly laundered pure cotton sheets (personally I prefer them to linen). I always remember asking a group of internationally recognized design gurus for their definition of real luxury and designer Sir Terence Conran came up with "river-washed linen sheets." He's not alone. Much of the Western world is getting awfully finicky about the sheets it sleeps in. Sophisticated shoppers want to know about fiber and thread counts, not to mention finish and esoteric little niche names.

Fellow linen fetishists may remember the widely hyped Sotheby's sale of the Duke and Duchess of Windsor's bed and table linen, which brought to the world's attention the charms of fine linen (theirs was from the French company of Porthault, as it happens) and every single piece was most beautifully and intricately embroidered with the Windsor cipher. Hot in its wake came a new kind of one-upmanship. The linen party hit the smarter reaches of New York, Washington, Chicago, and Los Angeles—an upmarket, more contemporary version of the old Tupperware do. The *New York Times* reported on the phenomenon with relish. Tales of women spending anything from $100 for a single pillowcase to $60,000 on closets full of bedding abounded. A sheet party was given for Annette Bening and Warren Beatty and some were even held at Gracie Mansion and at Blair House, the presidential guest house in Washington. "I would guarantee this is not about love-making," commented an etiquette expert (Clinton, you will have gathered, was still in office). "It's snobbery. It's for women who ask the ladies to lunch to see how their beds are made."

The sheet parties were the brainchild of one John Stoddart who had spent years working for one of New York's grandest linen shops (Leron, supplier to generations of Rockefellers as well as smart folk around the world) and who decided he could sell just as fancy linen but at rather lower prices by doing posh door to door. He sold the sort of sheets that made Fieldcrest and Ralph Lauren seem cheap. This was bed linen for those who wanted something that couldn't be found, as one of the partygoers put it, "on Bloomingdale's shelf." Madison Linens is possibly a bit on the fancy side for many tastes but those who'd like to check it out can visit the store at 1220 Broadway, New York 10001; 212-244-4380.

Hotels have now begun to realize that there's kudos (and therefore tony customers) to be had out of bed linen. Many now market themselves not just on the comfort of the rooms, the food and general hip quotient but also on the quality of the linen. The Lowell, one of New York's most charming small(ish) hotels mentions that it uses only Frette sheets high up in its marketing blurb. Frette ranks high in the pantheon of fine linen and is rumored to be the preferred brand of the Pope, Oprah, Brad Pitt and a host of others who can afford the $1,000 and more some of its sheets can cost.

At the Amanresorts, providers of sophisticated playgrounds for some of the world's richest and most spoiled travelers, it also has to be nothing but 100 percent pure Egyptian cotton. They can't name a brand because, as a spokesman put it, "our beds are so spacious that we have to get our linen specially made for us. But I can tell you that the crisp pure white Egyptian cotton looks so inviting on their own that we hardly ever use bedspreads."

The Mandarin Orientals in London and Hong Kong (where folklore has it that the sheets are ironed before night-time if a guest so much as sits on the bed during the day—it's all those creases, you see) use 100 percent Irish linen while the Ritz in Paris uses cotton percale from Porthault. Given not just the initial cost of the linen but the high maintenance, the laundry, and the ironing, it's all a powerful tribute to the greater sophistication and power of the traveling public.

Finally, here's a bit of advice that could only come out of America, and for which I am indebted to the *New York Times*: if you're thinking of having your linen monogrammed make sure to "monogram with your maiden name, so you'll get all the monogrammed bed linens in the divorce."

Where to Buy It

It's strange to think that it was for a time exceedingly hard to track down much in the way of white linen. Some fifteen years ago now a young girl working in the beauty department of U.K. *Harper's Bazaar* wanted to buy some white sheets for herself. She found that there wasn't a great deal of choice and so she came up with the idea of selling a range of white-only bed linen. I was the first person to write about it in the pages of the *Financial Times,* where I was an editor at the time. I thought it a great little idea. I had no idea that it would turn out to be a great *big* idea. She is now a multimillionairess—testimony to the power of white. These days **The White Company** (www.the whitecompany.com) sells much, much more than just a range of white linen—from blankets and linen clothing to a delectable collection of children's clothes its style is a hymn to all things pale and delicious. It will ship to the United States, although it may not make a great deal of financial sense, given the pound/dollar exchange rate and shipping charges—but if you can't find what you really want it could be worth checking out its collection online.

Personally I like my bed linen pure white but with a slightly vintage look (I love some white-on-white embroidery or lace), and so whenever I come upon some delicious new linen I snap it up. **Ardea Prime** goes in for rigorously plain linen sheets made from pure Irish linen—very austere, very beautiful, in white (from $185 for a single flat sheet)—and also has lots of other linen temptations (most particularly gorgeously elegant and unadorned damask tablecloths). Check them out at www.ardeaprime.com or call 248-598-1908.

Restoration Hardware (www.restorationhardware.com) has a lovely range, mostly white, some plain, some embroidered, some with lace, but also some pale stripes, some checks, and a few other colors.

Otherwise never forget **Bloomingdale's**. One of the nicest country houses I know, belonging to some close friends, has all its beds dressed entirely in linen from Bloomingdale's. Every time our friend visits New York she stocks up and the result is a delicious and varied collection of pure white linen, some plain, some embroidered, some embellished with lace. **Crate & Barrel** and **Pottery Barn** are two other great sources of classic bed linen. And on the shopping-center front, **Bed, Bath & Beyond** has some beautiful linens at very user-friendly prices.

TWO INSIDER ADDRESSES FOR LINEN FETISHISTS

Edith Mezard lives in the Château de l'Ange, in Lumières, not far from Avignon (+33 4 90 72 36 41). Hers is a favorite shop of both Princess Caroline of Monaco and Calvin Klein, and one can see why. Edith Mezard helps her husband run his haulage business in the morning and every afternoon, seven days a week, she opens up her shop. She sells beautiful old linens but also combines old and new textiles to create magic cushion covers, bedspreads, curtains. Almost every piece is different. There is hand-embroidered linen, plus a range of scented soaps, candles, and perfume for linen that rejoices in the name of Blanc, which, you may be sure, won't be in everybody else's linen closet back home.

Château de Bagnols, +33 4 74 71 40 00. If you're in the Beaujolais area, the shop attached to the hotel that Lady Hamlyn lovingly restored but which is now owned by the Von Essen group, sells many of the pieces that Lady Hamlyn commissioned exclusively for the chateau from a vast range of craftsmen, including finely embroidered linen sheets, damask tablecloths and lusciously beautiful towels with a discreet same-color (white) monogram.

Antique Linen

I've long had a fetish for antique linen, haring off down muddy roads in France at the smallest hint of a sign with the magic word, *brocantes*. What I think I'm going to do with it all, I can't imagine. Be that as it may, I now have several old monogrammed and embroidered sheets that make wonderful tablecloths, hand towels, and those heavy linen napkins that nobody seems to produce today. In old French market towns when they have their days selling *antiquités* or *brocantes,* you can still find antique pieces like this for very, very little. In the Sablon area of Brussels where there are some wonderful secondhand and antique shops, vintage linen for bed and table can often be found at excellent prices.

Jane Sacchi, whose appointment-only business at her house in London's Chelsea was for years a well-guarded secret among fellow linen fetishists, is now reachable by phone or e-mail (+44 20 7351 3160 or at www.janesacchi.com). She always has a supply of the finest monogrammed linen sheets (they also make terrific curtains), bold red-striped ticking, and hand-embroidered towels as well as bedspreads, tablecloths, tea towels, and pillowcases, often with the beautiful old monograms still intact. She also has a collection that is dyed a beautiful dusty old blue with the traditional woad or *bleus de pastel,* the dye that in the Middle Ages brought wealth to the towns of Albi and Toulouse. Prices aren't cheap—but then remember linen is almost forever—with single linen sheets starting at about $225.

The Lowdown on Thread Counts

Thread counts: a matter of great importance to the linen fetishist and increasingly cited by hotels to lure in picky customers (Schrager hotels, for instance, specify sheets with thread counts no lower than 350).

But there's no need to get too hung up on them. Thread counts refer to the number of strands in a square inch of sheeting. Generally speaking, the higher the thread count, the better and finer the sheets. However, most experts seem to agree that while the difference between a thread count of 120 and 250 matters greatly, once you go above 250 you're just showing off.

Besides thread counts, it's also finish that helps give a soft and silky feel. Frette, many experts agree, are among the finest of the fine (Gordon Campell Grey uses them in his impeccably chic hotels, No. 1 Aldwych and Carlisle Bay in Antigua), and much of the mystique is to do with the finish.

Fleur d'Andeol (check out www.fleurdandeol.com or call 646-291-8900 if you're looking for something not online) always has a mouthwatering selection of antique linen, including those deliciously traditional red and white tea towels and tablecloths. If the prices frighten you off, you can always settle for a lace handkerchief, monogrammed.

More on the Bedding Front

Silk duvets are a bit of an unknown luxury. Harry Kershaw, a latter-day merchant adventurer, imports from China some amazingly plain and beautiful pure silk duvets—that is, both the covers and the innards are all made entirely of silk, the covers of woven silk, the innards of silk floss. He's rather evangelical about them. To lie in bed under silk, he declares, is to sleep in the utmost luxury. The Eastern nobles (who cannily kept these indulgences for themselves) valued silk for its softness, warmth, and light weight. Sleeping under silk, they agreed, was rather "like being wrapped in a soft and delicate cloud." Its breathability, says Harry, enables it to absorb as much as 30 percent of its weight in moisture without feeling damp, and this keeps it feeling cool in summer yet warm in winter. It is also a boon to those who are allergic to some forms of bedding, for house mites, the cause of many allergies, do not, it seems, take to silk.

Duvets themselves generally come in two weights: 9 togs (a measure of its warmth) and 4½ togs. The idea is that most people would buy two—the lighter one for use in the summer, the heavier for use in autumn and spring, while in winter the two can be used together. At www.silkcomfort.com, prices range from $200 for a twin light silk duvet ($300 for a heavy version) and go on up to $325 for a king light ($475 for a heavy version).

BATHROOMS

I'm not going to talk here about the nitty-gritty of bathrooms: which bath to choose, which basin or which tap. Suffice it to say they can, and should, be glamorous, even in small spaces. One uses them all the time—certainly morning and evening—and they make a huge difference to one's morale. Even small ones can be made seductive if you keep them tidy and add candles, good mirrors (in fact, mirrors are a good way of creating glamour; a fantastic antique one, most particularly in a very modern bathroom, can soup up the look no end), divine soaps and oils. If you're sharing the bathroom, try to have two sinks. For busy people, it makes such a difference and cuts out all that business of two of you both trying to clean your teeth at the same time that goes on in the single-basin bathroom.

Babington House (I think) led the way in showing us that baths don't always have to be tucked away in closed-off bathrooms. There's something deeply seductive about a bath set in a wide window as an integral part of the bedroom. By taking away the need for a shut-off bathroom, a lot of space can be released to make the new bedroom-cum-bathroom infinitely airier.

If you haven't tried a proper shower you're missing out. These days there are fancy versions that imitate rainfall and offer all sorts of refinements but their main contribution to modern life is that it gets you in and out in record time and with minimum wastage of water.

Lovely fluffy towels—at least two sizes (one a big bath size and a smaller face size)—are essential and though they're more expensive than mean-sized, cheaper versions, they're not that much more expensive. It's not an economy worth making.

Neither is cheap soap. Fine, creamy, triple-milled soap isn't very much more expensive than cheap versions and yet it gives such a feeling of luxe in the bathroom. Buy a good make and enjoy it. Let me recommend as an occasional treat (rather than for every day) the wonderful pomegranate soap from the Farmaceutica di Santa Maria Novella in Florence (for details see page 156), but closer to home Jo Malone's soaps are beautiful too, as are those from Crabtree & Evelyn. I'm not a personal fan of those olive oil versions from Marseille (they're a bit too rough and *artisanal* for my taste), but plain unscented are pretty good. Ditto bath oils. We all have different notions of what smells great. I'm currently rather in love with Jo Woods's organic range, which is small, beautifully focused, smells divine (particularly her Usiku) and is entirely free of chemical nasties. I also love Ren's Moroccan Rose Otto with a passion. The point about bath oils, it seems to me, is that they're fabulous when they're really lovely but not worth having if they're not. Better to stick to water and a good soap if you can't afford something good.

The bathroom is also a great place to burn some delicious scented candles (see page 245).

KITCHENS

You can spend almost $100,000 on a kitchen without even trying (just check out the smart names such as Boffi, Bulthaup, and Varenna, with their fantastically seductive modern designs), but why would you? You get all sorts of fancy extras, it is true, like drawers that glide, a million different choices of internal arrangements and posh technical pyrotechnics (doors that fold swishly, extrawide drawers for storing saucepans, that sort of thing), but let me tell you that my own kitchen comes largely from Ikea. Our builder bought the cabinets (since Ikea makes them in their thousands, they can deliver terrific quality at rock-bottom prices) and then customized them to fit our space.

We live in an early Victorian house and the ground floor is a big open room—a dining area at the front and kitchen at the back—so the kitchen had to look good (as it can be seen from the dining table) and in keeping with the character of the house. I wanted it to be calm, rather like a cool Victorian larder or pantry, and unflashy. We've got built-in units on either wall that emulate the sort of huge dressers that you might have found in an old pantry and a large window at the back that overlooks lots of gardens. The only slightly luxurious touch is the cooktop, which is large (four burners and a central long range for a fish poacher plus two ovens). Otherwise we have a European-style fridge (I would have loved a huge upright one in stainless steel or sugar pink but there wasn't room), a dishwasher and lots of storage, as well as some open shelves on which we can display dishes and china.

The cornice, edgings, and woodwork are painted a very pale gray, while the main cabinet doors are painted a subtle greenish gray called Beauvais Gray, a shade I love. Our builder added grayish marble working surfaces, a little early Victorian molding to the cabinet doors and plain white china knobs. I love it and feel happy in it, and yet it cost relatively little.

The kitchen is now ten years old and if I were doing it again, I'd probably go more for stainless steel and lots of open shelving but there's something about having a restful kitchen, that isn't too trendy or edgy, that is very soothing as one softens an onion or stirs a sauce with some fabulous music playing all the while. If I had young children still around, I'd arrange things differently again and there would be a big kitchen table and old sofas to sink into, but as it is it does us beautifully.

I love old things such as antique creamy linen kitchen towels with that old-fashioned red stripe running through them. I collect them when I see them at fairs and in antique shops (Brussels if you happen to be going that way is a wonderful source). I also love those creamy bowls for mixing and all the classic old kitchen implements such as old glass cloches, cheese stands, vintage cutlery, enamel jugs, and bowls. I buy them when I see them at fairs and markets. There is something about them that has a long-lasting appeal—they've survived the test of time and give a much deeper pleasure than fancy, trendy, edgy kitchenware, which may amuse for a nanosecond but doesn't last the course. Crate & Barrel often has a nostalgic moment—just at the moment it's in a retro mood and there are some delicious ice-cream colored old-fashioned bowls and dishes, all of which have so much more appeal than anything too trendy or self-consciously fashionable.

LAUNDRY

There was a time when it looked as if Loving Hands were about to become the new Blahniks—i.e., a chic accessory for the yummy-mummy set. We haven't quite got there but the realization has now dawned that there are delicious cleaning materials around and that the nasty chemical varieties (though admittedly very efficient) that smell horribly of artificial compounds are no longer strictly necessary.

Ecover (www.ecover.com) is a new discovery in our household. The brand is sold in natural food stores (including Whole Foods) and has a whole raft of ecologically sound cleaning materials. More eco-friendly cleaning things like sponges and useful gadgets can be found at www.3rliving.com.

Cape Cod Lavender Farm (508-432-8397 and at www.capecodlavenderfarm.com) sells delicious little lavender pillows and sachets as well as a lavender linen spray.

The Laundress. For serious luxury I'm addicted to products from www.thelaundress.com. They're expensive but they smell more divine than any others I have come across. All their products have four basic scents: classic (citrus, ylang-ylang, and sandalwood); baby (vanilla, musk, bergamot, and lavender); cedar (perfect for woolens—cedarwood oil, frankincense, spices, and citrus zest); and lady (amber, citrus, and green herbs). Then there are products for whites, darks, baby clothes, linens, and cashmeres, as well as conditioners, ironing waters, stain solutions, and two amazing products called Crease Release (spray it on your linens and the creases fall out) and Stiffen Up (as effective as starch but smelling much nicer). Fabric Fresh is a spray for the upholstery that dogs, children, cigarette smoke, and the chaos of life have left smelling less than fresh. The Wool and Cashmere Shampoo (sulfate-free and smelling of cedar) is what they call the "hero" product: the one that, once tried, has a permanent place in the laundry cabinet. Prices are undoubtedly high but for the extra zing they add to the not-very-glamorous matter of doing the laundry I would reckon it worth it. They're mostly somewhere between $15 and $20, and the Wool and Cashmere shampoo is $18 and the Signature Detergent (for general laundering) is $19.50.

At the Laundress Web site, you can post your own laundry-related dilemmas to the girls. I posted mine, asking for help in getting red wine stains out of the white tablecloths I love and which our local laundry never seems to deal with (though it is highly skilled at folding the cloths so that you don't notice the stain is still there until you get it home). I sent my e-mail at about four P.M. and had a reply by nine P.M. In case you have the same problem, this is it:

> Hello, Lucia,
>
> Ah, the downfall of the fabulous red wine. We wouldn't launch our products until we were able to conquer red wine and yellow armpit stains.

This is my method for red wine.

In a sink or bin, pour the Laundress Stain Solution directly onto the wine stain and rinse with HOT water. Repeat, repeat, repeat. The wine first turns gray, then yellowish.

When I get to the yellowish state I launder (with hot water) with our Whites Detergent and pour extra detergent on the remaining spot. Do not put in the dryer if the spot is still visible. Re-wash as the dryer will set in the stain. Successful on my white linen slipcovers, too many times than I'd like.

Happy Laundering!

To liven up the laundry room, Cath Kidston (cathkidston.com) does the cheeriest of covers for the ironing-board and, to save on all that table linen (this is for those who have children or grandchildren), she does wonderfully pretty plastic cloths that you just wipe clean.

FLOWERS

As I've already remarked, I've often thought that the things that really matter in a house (apart from it being filled with people one loves—the one true necessity) are books, flowers, music, food and wine, none of which need be expensive. San Franciscans who can muster the energy to get up early can buy huge boxes full of flowers at the Flower Mart (in the SoMa district) for very, very little—and you don't have to be there *that* early (anything up to eight-thirty A.M. is fine). Stores such as Macy's and Nordstrom are getting much better on the taste front, and what I call their "arrangements" are getting less pretentious and more attractive by the day.

The rules set down by the old Constance Spry school of floristry ("Always form a triangle," and "Never have even numbers of anything" were two unchanging mantras) are mostly outmoded, though the looser, more ephemeral sort of unwritten rules are more difficult to follow.

> ☛ *Remember, you can put flowers into a whole variety of containers that aren't officially labeled vases. Huge glass jugs, or old milk jugs in country houses look wonderful, as do ice cream bowls, little ceramic holders, coffee cups, tumblers, or even old tins—use your imagination.*

For those who like rules—and they do, after all, simplify the matter—hang on to this one: if in doubt, never mix your flowers. Just have masses and masses of one thing, the more you can afford the better. Were you to be so misguided as to put some hyacinths with roses, or tulips together with daffodils or—worse—combine tulips with orchids, ooh, goodness, I can feel the taste police shuddering now. You can—just to complicate the matter—combine certain flowers (this is where personal eye and taste are everything) but experts agree that you should then stick with a one- or two-color palette, for example whites and lime greens and creams, or pinks and reds, or lilacs and blues.

For somebody who isn't into the artless and romantic, and wants something on the chic side, florist Nikki Tibbles uses what she calls "gorgeous wax vases" and for, say, a dinner party, she might suggest planting them down the middle of a table filled with "a hedge of lilac roses." The roses should be cut quite short so that the heads are just over the top of the vase, and here she gives a useful tip: "The taller the stem, the fatter the rose head, so you'll need fewer of them." Another Nikki Tibbles tip: change the water daily.

At Marston & Langinger's brilliant newly expanded showroom at 192 Ebury Street, London SW1W 8UP (www .marston-and-langinger.com), Simon Lycett, who looks after all the flowers, comes with a little bit of provenance since he did the flowers for *Four Weddings and a Funeral,* which we all got to have a gander at, and for the wedding of Posh and Becks, which we did not, as well as for Elton John's fiftieth birthday party. Peter and Susan Marston (of the Marston part of the name) are great proponents of simplicity. "Contorted willow is a big no-no. No weeping willow, either. And no cruelty to plants and certainly no floral bondage. Little wire spikes to hold them together or string that is too tight are another big no-no. Gerberas—no. Carnations—no." And those once oh-so-chic zinc containers that all the Milanese florists use are very much a no, too. No mixtures: "They come from the gas station school of floristry."

So what rates a yes? Purple hyacinths—so beautiful that you can just stick them in an empty paint tin. A huge moss cushion of massed white crocuses looks great. ("How do you water it?" I asked rather mundanely; "You sprinkle it," came the reply—but then practicality, as Peter Marston put it, isn't what flowers are about.) Great big blowsy pale pink peonies are very much yes: "When the petals drop just let them lie there—they're perfection." The "straight from the greenhouse look" is very in—just take things like fritillaries in terracotta pots straight to the table. Little tiny pots of grass, especially wheatgrass, look wonderful, all bright green and neatly clipped.

Ercoli of McQueens, who does the *Vanity Fair* party at the Oscars (126 St. John Street, London EC1V 9AN; +44 20 7251 5505), is also of the simple school of floristry. "I hate formulas," he says, "and I hate mixtures. I just love lots and lots of bulbs and the sense of smell is important—have a great rosemary plant in the kitchen, for instance, or in the bedroom and bathroom have big groups of snowdrops or daffodils. Simple things like leaves and stones look good, too."

If you have the sort of home that sports cutting-edge B & B Italia furniture, clean minimalist lines, lots of cream, gray, and black—you get the picture—then probably you are in need of what these days are called "flower designers." In the U.K. Robert Hornsby, the creative spirit behind a company called Inwater (check some of his designs on www.inwater.uk.com), is the leading proponent of the trend. He made his name by submerging flowers under water (hence the name). Nowadays this is thought a bit passé, though to be truthful I still sometimes find this ravishing (one of Robert Hornsby's tricks was—and sometimes is—to color both flower and water with fabric dyes). He likes great big torpedo-style shapes and will sink flowers underwater on stones, or lots of just one flower crammed inside a very clean-cut container. He's also fond of big "bombs" (perhaps in these nervy days a happier term might be "domes") of massed roses or arum lilies. He likes to use fluorescent lime-green Perspex underneath a flower arrangement to give it a subliminal glow. All these can—if you have the will and the eye—be copied at home.

Cutting-edge florists in the United States who do this sort of thing are www.thedesignersco-op.com and you can have a peep at their taste by checking into their Web site.

I think nothing is nicer than country roses, from the garden rather than forced greenhouse ones, and you can get them in season, of course, from Ashdown Roses (877-274-3696 and at www.ashdownroses.com), a flower farm in the foothills of the Blue Ridge Mountains.

There you have it: it's not rocket science, just a question of keeping it simple.

How to Make Flowers Last

1. Cut the stems off shop-bought flowers at an angle as you soon as you get them home.

2. Always use a very clean vase.

3. Keep the water clean. A drop of bleach will help keep the water sterilized and so stop the stems from rotting.

4. An ice cube in the vase helps revive flowers that are wilting.

5. Use the plant food the florist provides, but if you're cutting your own, add some sugar.

SCENTED CANDLES

You may be of the school of thought that hates them. I love them when they're wonderful but when they're bad, they're horrid. I'm unashamedly picky about them and like only the best and most expensive, because I'd rather the house smelled of fresh coffee, fresh flowers and simple honest soap than cheaply scented candles. And just so you know my prejudices, I don't like them sweet and floral either. With a (very) few exceptions I like them spicy, rich, mysterious. I also learned from Jo Malone that you can create something new by burning two at once—amber and lavender, for instance, smell divine when burned together but there are lots of other combinations to try. Valentine Alexander, my makeup guru, always burns Diptyque's Figuier and Menthe Verte at the same time.

So here's my list of great scented candles. It's personal, idiosyncratic, and very, very picky.

Rigaud, the French candles that come in glass containers with a little metal saucer, are for me the all-time winner—subtle, sophisticated, classy. They remind me of those French apartments with an enfilade of elegant rooms, each one lightly perfumed, as well as those grand Park Avenue apartments with dark-red lacquered walls and toffee-varnished floors. Cypres, a light smell of wood and pines, is my favorite, but there's also Cendre, Cythère, and Tournesol. Find them in chic stores such as Bergdorf Goodman, in little boutiques with taste, and in London at Thomas Goode (19 South Audley Street, London W1K 2BN; +44 20 7499 2823; www.thomasgoode.co.uk).

Lorenzo Villoresi is a Florentine (of noble birth—what else?) who seems to spend his days like a mediaeval alchemist, sniffing, stirring, and mixing potions and lotions in a Florentine aerie. His scents are rich, mysterious, sensual, and addictive. Rumor has it that Cherie Blair took some of his scents as a house present when staying with the Queen at Balmoral. He makes custom perfumes from the finest oils and essences and uses only natural fixes. I like best his Sandalwood and his Spezie, but almost all of them are lovely. Best of all, make an appointment to go to his aerie at 12/14 Via de' Bardi, 50125 in Florence (you'll have to call first: +39 05 5234 1187) and sniff for yourself. Otherwise, Lafco NY (212-925-0001; www.lafcony.com) stocks his wares, as well as rather select boutiques around the world, including Fortnum & Mason (+44 20 7734 8040) and Les Senteurs (71 Elizabeth Street, London SW1W 9PJ; +44 20 7730 2322)

Diptyque does gorgeous scents, something like fifty of them. From Madonna (Figeur and Verveine) and Puff Daddy (Tuberose) to Nigella Lawson (Rose) and Elizabeth Hurley (Figeur), the line has many fans. I don't like them all, but I'm mad about a few, most particularly Figuier. Don't be afraid to burn a couple of candles together. Visit their boutique in San Francisco (171 Maiden Lane, San Francisco 64108; 415-402-0600) or you can find Diptyque in many places, such as Space NK and Neiman Marcus.

Ormonde Jayne, a delectable little shop in the Royal Arcade, off Old Bond Street (+44 20 7499 1100 and at www.ormondejayne.com—and she's going to be coming soon to New York), has a small but distinguished and growing cult following. Allegra Hicks is a great fan, as is Anoushka Hempel, who buys her candles in Pink Grapefruit by the fistful. Another customer, who heads up a posh luxury goods company in Old Bond Street, comes in every Saturday morning and buys four of her Green Tea candles (I can't quite make out whether he's got a lot of homes or a single house with a lot of rooms, but we have to hope he's got good fire insurance). Green Tea smells like a smoky Lapsang Souchong, very refined, very delicious, while Pink Grapefruit is crisper.

Jo Malone (www.jomalone.com). It still takes a lot to beat her Amber and Sweet Orange scented candle and if you're feeling extravagant at Christmas you could burn a giant-sized one with four wicks. I love her Grapefruit, her Wild Fig and Cassis, and her Pomegranate Noir. Her candles make a terrific present. You can order from 866-305-4706.

If you're giving a party it adds to the magic if you burn lots of little candles. Try something like Penhaligon's miniature candles in fresh, green-smelling Lavandula (www.penhaligons.com).

☞ *Remember to trim the wick each time before you light candles. Long wicks flop over and tend to disappear into the molten wax. Scented candles don't, I think, mix well with food, so keep them out of the dining room. And colored candles (in my view) aren't great—keep them white, cream, or black (which is quite sensual somehow).*

DECLUTTERING

Most people's response to having too much stuff is to think they need more closet space. In fact the problem lies in having too much stuff. Get rid of some of it. The hard bit is finding the will to do it. Because nobody is going to die if you leave it for another day, it's awfully tempting to say, oh sod it, it can wait. If you're a sod-it sort of person, there are clutter counselors (yes, really; even Madonna has been known to call on their services) to help put you right. There is also the more practical breed of person who will order files, stick photographs in albums, arrange your DVDs and get rid of the papers you don't need. It does, unfortunately, involve a bit of decluttering of the bank account but it's probably worth it.

I have a friend who was in such a bad way that she could scarcely find the teapot in the mornings. She'd screwed up the place with belongings, all of which had played some emotional role in her life. She called in a clutter consultant, who certainly caused her to shed some tears (she is rather sentimental, my friend; she's had several marriages and many *affaires du coeur* and everything reminded her of somebody), but who also got her sorted out.

This kind of service might seem as if it were geared to the idle rich but it's mostly used by busy professional women who find themselves overwhelmed by conflicting demands. They're just people in a muddle. Some of them were living amid such clutter that they were ashamed to ask friends home. Sometimes it's just a matter of being shown how to make proper files, when to throw out old checkbooks (it's certainly not worth keeping them for more than five years), or getting help with organizing photographs into albums. If you work at home, or are suddenly changing from an office life to a home-based working life, she'll help you set up an efficient home office.

There are clutter gurus across the country who can help (go to www.napo.net to find an organizer in your area). "Many people," said one professional organizer, "just don't seem to know how much paperwork to keep and how much to throw out. We'll come in, look at your files, help work out a proper system for you and then put it all in order. Usually it shouldn't take more than two or three days to sort somebody's paperwork."

If you've got young children or a baby, it's worth knowing that there are shops across the country where mothers have a sort of exchange system going where they buy and sell things like high chairs, strollers, cots, tricycles, and the like. They buy when they need them and sell when they've finished with them. The profits usually go to needy children and families.

Small Things That Help

1. Try to keep untidiness at bay by doing a little as you go. Once things get really out of hand and a major effort is required, it becomes too dispiriting.

2. If you have children, get some attractive boxes (wicker ones are particularly nice) that fit under shelves. It makes it easy to sweep toys into them in one easy movement.

3. Small baskets or attractive trays and boxes can be used to order cosmetics and jewelry.

4. Jewelry can be stored decoratively. I've seen a wall covered with decorative hooks around which necklaces, bracelets, and the like were draped.

5. If you can keep surfaces clear, it helps to provide an aura of calm.

Do It Yourself

Life's too precious to spend time searching for things.
—Dawna Walter

It goes without saying that if you can face sorting your files and office on your own, it'll be a lot cheaper. You could start, though, by buying Dawna Walter's book *Life Laundry: How to De-Junk Your Life* ($15) and scouring it for tips. She always maintains that nobody, except the extremely leisured, can afford the time to be disorganized or to have too much clutter. If you can lay your hand on what you need the minute you need it, she believes you can save several hours a week.

Muji (455 Broadway, New York 10013; 212-334-2002; www.muji.com) for files and storage. It doesn't have a large selection but what it has is brilliant. There are elegant, transparent boxes of almost every size and shape (great for organizing cosmetics, too) as well as transparent files that cost very little.

Target is fabulous for inexpensive storage. If you're really short of space, you can get a set of six clear sliding boxes, which can be slotted away under the bed.

The Container Store's raison d'être is providing storage solutions and it has them to fit almost every aesthetic: steely, baskety, pastel. Call 888-266-8246 for a catalog or go to www .containerstore.com.

My Great Home, at www.mygreathome.com is a wonderful source of storage advice.

Any Junk: Charity shops will take good things but not chipped china, shabby clothes, broken toys and knickknacks. For a fee, 1-800-GOT-JUNK? will come and take all your discarded junk away. Go to www.1-800-got-junk.com or call 800-468-5865.

iSold It (www.i-soldit.com and 1-888-916-1110) will sell your unwanted things on eBay—for a fee.

Your local government will often take away unwanted junk for a small fee. Larger branches of many supermarkets have big bins where you can dump your rejected shoes, books, clothing and other castoffs. For clearing up the mess in your garden, for example, look in the Yellow Pages under removals and you'll find tons of companies ranging from huge outfits to a man with a van.

www.freecycle.org is the Web site of an organization dedicated to recycling or giving away unwanted goods so that they don't go to waste. You can give your own unwanted stuff away as well as find things you may need.

Pods (866-229-4120 and at www.pods.com). And finally, if you're really unable to "let go" or own, say, family stuff you really shouldn't "let go," there is always a storage company that will store it for you.

☞ *Remember: tidiness matters but only to a degree. It's not more important than having time for your family, playing with your children, cooking lovely meals or reading a good book. Comfort yourself with the fact that it was Le Corbusier, that great rationalist and minimalist, who admitted that order isn't everything: "Life always has the last word." Remember, too, the poet Andrew Marvell's words: "The grave's a fine and private place. But none, I think, do there embrace." Think of that as you gaze at the mess and you'll feel a whole lot better.*

CHEAP CHIC

Unless you have a feeling for that secret knowledge that modest things can be more beautiful than anything expensive, you will never have style.

—ANDRÉE PUTMAN

The problem with furnishing on a shoestring is that to do it brilliantly requires immense ingenuity. I once read of a New York restaurant owner who put hand-sanded acrylic mirror, a quarter of an inch thick, on the floor of his restaurant at a cost of just $6 per square foot—whoever would have thought of that? (In case you're interested, it's available from Industrial Plastic Supply at 309 Canal Street, New York 10013 (212-226-2010.)

Otherwise it takes time, energy, and taste buds that are more than usually alert. Pick up, say, the Sears catalog and, in among stuff that you wouldn't give house room to, you will find some gems. Pass over the sickly bedding with beaded stars and the faux-naif patchworks, and home in on the slinky bath fittings: fashionably shaped pedestal basins in glass or plain white ceramic at a fraction of the prices to be found in swanky bathroom shops. Check out the chrome fittings—avoid the curlicues and go for the plain shelves and towel holders, and you could save yourself a fortune. Lighting too. Look out for well-priced bedroom furniture, painted white with simple wooden handles, and some ready-made, plain, tab-headed curtains in simple cottons or silks (www.sears.com).

If, like my son and his wife after they bought a farmhouse in the Cévennes, you need to set out a large number of beds (at least twelve in their case) in a hurry it's worth looking at The Company Store (www.thecompanystore.com). It has plain sheets in pure cotton in a range of mouth-watering colors (including white, pale blue, sage green, sand, and ivory) at absurdly low prices. While Ikea can probably beat its prices, Ikea doesn't do what The Company Store does: take orders by phone and deliver to the door.

Well-priced lighting comes from Home Depot, and Crate & Barrel. Ikea, if you can face the schlep, is good on inexpensive lighting. Ikea is also fabulous for inexpensive shelving, bookcases, and the like.

If you're looking for dishware you could scarcely do better than Crate & Barrel, which has some thankfully plain white china at very good prices. Otherwise go to www.KlinQ.com, where you can buy simple white catering crockery (almost childproof) in bulk. And there are all manner of plain white porcelain soufflé and baking dishes at equally beguiling prices. For something a little prettier—some charming pale aqua-green bowls, for instance—Muji is pretty good, too.

It's much better, when it comes to things like curtains, to be generous with less expensive fabrics (oceans of calico or canvas can look wonderful, and you can add borders to make them look bespoke) than to be mean with expensive ones. Curtains should always trail a bit on to the floor.

Otherwise scour Indian shops for saris. Now that houses are starting to be softened up again, saris, draped over curtain rings, make ravishingly pretty curtains. (Before I redid our drawing room, which is now curtainless, our curtains were made from twelve white-on-white appliquéd bedspreads bought for $10 each in Udaipur.)

If you're tempted by the Conran Shop's offerings but find the prices beyond you, check out their semi-annual warehouse sales—but be sure to be there early, as inevitably all of the best things are snatched up instantly.

As I write, what is known as "brown furniture" is going for rock-bottom prices. The mood is for the new, the edgy, the avant-garde. It's the loft-living set and the hedge-fund guys who've set the pace and they all want new, new, new. This means that those who like antique furniture can buy it at wonderful prices. Country auctions are a good source of inexpensive pieces. Check the local papers where you live as most areas have an auction house not too far away. Antique shops are obviously good sources if you have a good eye but they take energy and persistence. I love snooping around the Golborne Road in London's North Kensington where there is a whole series of good shops selling inexpensive French country furniture, mirrors, fireplaces and other decorative pieces. I once found four Charlotte Perriand steel and leather chairs for around $600 in a shop in the Golborne Road. (Charlotte Perriand was a wonderful designer and design fundis will know she used to work with Le Corbusier.)

And don't forget the sales. A white sink is a white sink and it's no less desirable because it's being sold off at a cheaper price. I've already mentioned that we always replace our Riedel glasses (rather expensive, beautifully austere, unadorned wine glasses) in an annual sale. Soap is another good thing to buy discounted.

When it comes to floors, remember that there's scarcely anything nicer than painted floorboards (even old ones can be renovated with some sanding and the flaws are part of their charm), while sea-grass matting is relatively inexpensive and very attractive. Instead of Persian rugs or handwoven silks think of using a rug of sea-grass matting edged with a wide border in chocolate (or some other neutral color).

Cheap collections of things—even chandeliers or furniture—can be given a bit of pizzazz by painting them chalky white. I've seen touristy African masks transformed by painting a group of them in chalky white; they immediately looked intriguing and chic.

☛ *Instead of throwing out furniture because it looks shabby, think of recycling it. Give it new life by painting it matte black or chalky gray-white, or lacquer the surface in deep vermilion, black, or scarlet. Sofas or chairs that look old can be given a bit of new life by a great throw, which is much cheaper than reupholstering.*

If you're short of money, though, the real pitfall to avoid is buying anything you don't really, really love. I know, I know, sometimes it is unavoidable. I remember well moving into our first house when we were very poor (we were about to produce a baby and had just taken on what for us was a vast mortgage) and all of a sudden we needed carpeting for four floors plus the stairs, as well as—if I remember correctly—something like twenty-seven light fittings. We bought loop carpeting and Japanese paper lights. They were just about all right but I never liked either much and so, in due course, we replaced the paper lights and the carpeting for something better. In other words the money we first spent was really wasted. If we'd bought slowly one by one things we really loved, we wouldn't have had to replace anything at all.

Common things, everyday things
are the most important things.
—Margaret Visser

If you are short of money, take comfort from the thought that throwing money at the problem doesn't always result in a nicer, more interesting house. On the contrary, very often this can make a house look cold and overdesigned, too perfect. All the best houses take years to evolve, layer upon layer. That gives them depth and interest. As the years roll by they become a living archive, bearing witness to the history of the house and the stories of those who live in it. No interior decorator with their instant solutions, their bulging address books and professional know-how could ever create a house as interesting, as particular and as individual as the houses that are truthful expressions of their owners and the lives they've lived. Those who are short of money have to make their houses more personal, hunt for bargains, improvise a bit, but this gives character and individuality. And money was never, anyway, any guarantee of taste.

Room Doctors

Just as I'm a fan of personal shoppers—they can winkle out a whole new side of one's personality or show one ways of dressing that one hadn't thought of—so I'm rather a fan of getting professional advice on the interiors front. The thing about professionals is that they do what they do all the time. They've dealt with a million narrow passageways, kitchen-dining rooms or first-floor, L-shaped drawing rooms, and have sussed out how to make them work. Those of us who move house occasionally and have other jobs don't get enough practice at solving the practical problems. Getting it wrong on the interiors front (moving the wrong wall, for instance; making a silly decision about where to put the coatroom or the kitchen; not plotting the lighting scheme soon enough) is a very expensive business. I've never been able to afford the whole first-class expensive interior design service (which, anyway, as we saw earlier, I think leads to too impersonal a result) but I have found that buying bits of expertise pays off hands down.

In the last five years we've been redoing our house floor by floor as it had got very shabby and out of date. Just as we were about to embark on trying to do the drawing room, I heard about Christopher Prain and Chanond Purananda, a couple of young interior designers who were just starting in the business. For a small commission on the expenditure they agreed not only to come up with ideas (which we would obviously have to approve) but—fantastically—to organize it all. I loved their ideas—they "got" my slightly boho, eclectic tastes perfectly—and once that was agreed they organized the removal men (because we had to empty the room completely if the builders were to meet the two-week deadline that we'd given them) and the sending of the discarded pieces to Christie's.

They brought to my attention fabrics, furniture and ideas that I hadn't thought of or known about. Chanond suggested a brilliant deep apple-green paint for the inside of the bookshelves. I would never, ever have come up with that myself and yet I love it. It's very, very glamorous. They suggested a subtle wallpaper from Knowles & Christou (or Stark Carpet in the United States) as well its Lulu cabinet with delicately pretty painted glass fronts to house the TV. Everybody falls in love with it. They found an antique iron cot at Alfie's Antique Market (see page 258) and turned it into a small sofa. Together we trawled the antique markets and found a wonderful 1930s photographer's light and a nicely shabby French 1930s leather armchair. We added another light, by Flos, and a small Eileen Grey table. They tracked down the perfect rugs—one from Christine van der Hurd, which she just happened to have in stock, and one, in deep olive green with delicate purple swirls, which was specially woven in Nepal, from Veedon Fleece. They created a very beautiful screen, which is printed with fine copies of a hand-engraved map done by John Rocque and published in 1746 (see it on www.motco.com), and it's set into a black-lacquered frame. I think it's wonderful.

Working with professional designers has reaffirmed my belief that not only does it ease the whole burden (they made sure that finishes were right, that builders turned up on time; they helped make decisions about light switches and door handles), *but* even more importantly they widened the scope, offering ideas and solutions that I'd never have had on my own.

Yes, it did cost more than we'd envisaged but on the other hand it is infinitely more exciting than our modest plan would have left it. Given that we hadn't done anything for twenty years, it seems like money well spent.

I used Christopher Chanond Designs who work out of 66A Tachbrook St., London SW1V 2NA (+44 20 7630 1155 and at www.christopherchanond.com). They will give advice by the hour (at about $200 an hour) or will do the design work for you but let you find your own builder and project manage it yourself. Alternatively, they can do this on your behalf, in which case they charge 10 percent of the cost of the project. If they just source suitable items, they take a small handling charge on the furniture and goods they buy, but this is at trade cost and they don't charge the customer the full retail price so there's always a saving for the clients. Other people I know recommend a Washington practice called Cole Prevost (1635 Connecticut Ave. NW, Washington, D.C. 20009; 202-234-1090).

There are small design practices all over the country that can offer a similar service but clearly the quality of the advice varies—there's nothing like seeing their work and asking around among your friends. You can also get design advice from quite a lot of companies that specialize in selling furniture and furnishings. For instance, Laura Ashley (whose home collection is filled with little gems in my view—they're not avant-garde or edgy but they are charming and very usable), offers design advice free.

Most kitchen companies will design kitchens for no charge.

Alfie's Antique Market, 13–25 Church St., London NW8 8DT (+44 20 7233 6066 and at www.alfiesantiques.com) and its sister market, Grey's, 58 Davies St., London W1K 5A8 (+44 20 7629 7304 and at www.greysantiques.com), both have personal shoppers to help track down the things you'd like. Since I think they have some of the best selection of charming, decorative antiques in London (particularly if you're looking for a suitably shabby armchair or a stunning light), this could be well worth doing. It's by appointment only—call +44 20 7725 9601. You can find similar services in New Orleans to trawl the markets in the French Quarter and on Market Street.

Favorite Shops Around the World

Here is a list of my favorite shops, the ones I snoop around when in need of something new or just to be inspired. I have to apologize for the fact that most of them are in London but that is where I live and so it's the place I know best. Several have Web sites, though, so you can access their products wherever you are.

CUTTING EDGE AND CONTEMPORARY

Aram, 110 Drury Lane, London WC2B 5SG (+44 20 7240 3933 and at www.aram.co.uk). The place for the grand twentieth-century classics—Shiro Kuramata, Eileen Grey (whom Zeev Aram rediscovered and for which Aram is the official licensee), Breuer and many more, but there are lots of funky, avant-garde pieces as well.

Mint, 70 Wigmore Street, London W1U 2SF (+44 20 7224 4406 and at www.mintshop.co.uk). This is tiny but is on every design aficionado's list of regular places to drop into. You might find some delicate handmade ceramics from an innovative new designer, some glorious rococo transparent resin mirrors, a mad chandelier, some papier-mâché Chinese urns or some classic French pottery, not to mention Maarten Baas's wonderfully edgy smoked furniture. (His technique is to take existing pieces and "burn" them—yes, really—and lest you think this is a joke let me tell you that the renowned Li Edelkoort got him to burn her grand piano.)

The Conran Shop, Michelin House, 81 Fulham Rd., London SW3 6RD (+44 207 589 7401—it also has a shop at 407 East Fifty-ninth Street, New York 10022; 212-755-9079—and at www.conranusa.com). The first stop for those checking out what's latest, new, and hot. It's expensive but keeps one up to speed. The mix has been livened up in recent times with some vintage finds—a Victorian shirt cabinet from an old shop, French farmhouse tables—placed next to a wildly cutting-edge glass table with curvy scarlet legs. Great for presents: toys for the boys, gadgets, tableware, design books, delicious smellies, and food.

TwentyTwentyOne, 274 Upper Street, London N1 2UA and 18C River St., London EC1R 1XN (+44 20 7288 1996 and at www.twentytwentyone.com). *The* shops for fine reeditions of the great twentieth-century classics—Breuer's Wassily chair, the Barcelona, Le Grand Confort, the Corbusier chaise longue, Eileen Grey, et al. But also lots of fun small things from watches to lighting to kitchenware.

MORE GALLERY THAN SHOP

David Gill, 60 Fulham Road, London SW3 6HH (+44 20 7589 5946) and 2 Loughborough Street, London SE11 5RP (+44 20 7793 1100). Gill is part shopkeeper, part gallery owner, part collector and curator. He specializes in twentieth-century decorative objects and mixes grand classic designs with very avant-garde work by our finest artists and craftsmen. He's been responsible for introducing a host of designers to the British—from Garouste and Bonetti (when they were a working partnership) to Oriel Harwood. Very expensive but absolutely fascinating.

Rabih Hage, 69–71 Sloane Avenue, London SW3 3DH (+44 20 7823 8288 and at www.rabih-hage.com). The place to see radical design. He often uncovers new designers before anybody else has got to them. There's always a fascinating exhibition—the last one was on recycled furniture, while others have homed in on weirdly beautiful lights by Gaetano Pesce that look more like invertebrates than lamps. Hage has a fine eye and it is the place for really original pieces.

Themes & Variations, 231 Westbourne Grove, London W11 25E (+44 20 7727 5531 and at www.themesandvari ations.com). A large and airy gallery-cum-shop with lights-cum-sculpture and pieces by Fornasetti. In all an eclectic mix of original, beautiful things that are halfway between functional items and art.

Vessel, 114 Kensington Park Road, London W11 2PW (+44 20 7727 8001 and at www.vesselgallery.com). This has very innovative ceramics, featuring designs by Hella Jongerius, Ted Muehling, Marcel Wanders, and other darlings of the avant-garde design world. Always beautiful, always interesting.

QUIRKY SPECIALISTS

Abigail Aherne, 137 Upper Street, London N1 1QP (+44 20 7354 8181). A delicious shop whose owner just seems to buy what takes her fancy. Her style is what you might call boho-eclectic: flocked anglepoise lights, gorgeous rugs, quirky accessories.

After Noah, shops at 261 King's Road, London SW3 5EL (+44 20 7351 2610), and 121 Upper Street, London N1 1QP (+44 20 7359 4281), and at www.afternoah.com. A good source of old classics, from old American hospital furniture to classic lights. Usually lots of anglepoise lights, old enamelware, school desks, Shaker-style children's chairs, old cupboards—what is commonly known as eclectic but great for a good rummage.

Nicole Farhi Living, 17 Clifford Street, London W15 2VE (+44 20 7494 9051). If you can't get to the Paris flea markets, Nicole Farhi does it for you—at a price. A wonderfully enchanting mix of French flea-market finds: worn leather chairs, library steps, eglomise glass-topped tables, exquisite ceramics, deliciously scented candles, huge glass bell jars and anything else that takes the very clever eye of the buyer.

Labour and Wait, 18 Cheshire Street, London E2 6EH (+44 20 7729 6253 and at www.labourandwait.co.uk). A cult shop that goes in for sturdy brooms and brushes, enamelware, tinware, all the old-fashioned household equipment that our grandmothers were supposed to have used, brown paper, sturdy string and rope, old-fashioned glass.

GREAT FOR ANTIQUES

Guinevere Antiques, 574–580 King's Road, London SW6 2DY (+44 20 7736 2917 and at www.guinevere.co.uk). One of the most beautiful antique shops in London—but *very* expensive. Beautiful old Tang clay figures, fine old French linen, antique silver, crystal glasses. Whatever is beautiful, whether from China, French provincial chateaux, Italian villas and palazzos, or the grand old houses of England, the Guinevere buyers pick out the very best.

Judy Greenwood, 657–659 Fulham Rd., London SW6 5PY (+44 20 7736 6037 and at www.judygreenwoodantiques .co.uk). She specializes in French provincial charm, laid on thick. For anything from a magic little chandelier or a range of old enamel kitchen tins to a great big kitchen dresser.

DEPARTMENT STORES

Liberty, Regent St., London W1B 5TR (+44 20 7734 1234). A wonderfully eclectic collection of furniture with some fine old vintage pieces—some very old (an amazingly shabby eighteenth-century chair, for instance), some mid-twentieth-century classics and some spanking new and exciting modern pieces, such as the very experimental work of the newly launched cooperative Established and Sons. Liberty also has the only outlet in the U.K. for the designs of Svensk Tenn, the famous Swedish purveyors of Josef Franck's vibrant fabrics and small pieces of furniture.

UNITED STATES

Crate & Barrel (www.crateandbarrel.com), I always look in on Crate & Barrel whenever I'm in America—it has a high standard of design, and I like its atmosphere. It has fantastically desirable pieces and, besides its well-priced furniture (I remember seeing gorgeously shabby leather furniture long before it was easily available anywhere else), lots of small things such as china, candlesticks, glass, and so on that are pretty easy to pack.

Pottery Barn (www.potterybarn.com) does lots of things well but I was most struck but its vast range of inexpensive cutlery in every mood and style (resin, wood, steel, silver, glass, and bamboo) as well as inexpensive huge plain white heavy linen catering tablecloths (very hard to find anywhere else), candlesticks, and linen.

Williams-Sonoma (www.williams-sonoma.com) is quite simply the best cook's shop in the world. Whether you're after some esoteric ingredients, a retro food-mixer in a delectable color or the sharpest, most long-lasting knives, Williams-Sonoma will have it.

All three of these shops have branches all over the States. **Bloomingdale's** linen department, as I've already pointed out, is a joy. After that I head down to SoHo where **Murray Moss**'s eponymous emporium, at 150 Greene Street, New York 10012, is a design mecca (www.mossonline.com; 866-888-6677). If you want a contemporary overview of all that's best and happening in design you can't do better than call in at Murray Moss. In the surrounding streets there are always new funky, design-led stores to check out. I always check up on **Shabby Chic** at 83 Wooster Street, New York 10012; 212-274-9842, which goes in for the sort of slightly faded boho look that I'm so fond of. **ABC Carpet & Home** (888 Broadway, New York 10003; 212-473-3000; www.abchome.com) is a New York classic, a wonderfully eclectic amalgam of different tastes and moods. It's great obviously for carpets but also for all those small things—cushions, door handles, lamps, small antiques—that do for a house what accessories do for an outfit.

CITE, 131 Greene Street, New York, does a wonderful mix of established modern names (Eero Aarnio, Verner Panton), funky avant-garde, and anything old that catches the buyers' eyes. Matter, 405 Broome Street, SoHo, New York, and 227 Fifth Avenue, Brooklyn, New York, are great shops for design fundis. Interesting furniture but also good for presents—small lamps, mirrors, key-rings, jewelry, ceramics and strange *objets*.

PARIS

Paris is no longer as cheap as it was, but if you're furnishing from scratch or just looking for a few very decorative pieces, it's fun to go and do it there. Go on a Friday (many shops in Paris are closed on Mondays), stay in a small left-bank hotel (saving your euros for the temptations that lie ahead) and then plan your days like a military campaign.

Keep a day for the left bank and a wander around the rue Jacob and the Place St. Sulpice, another day for the Marais, and at least a morning for the great unmissable treat of a good rummage around the flea market at the Porte de Clignancourt.

The Left Bank

Modénature, 3 rue Jacob, Paris 75006; +33 1 53 10 31 70. Modénature sells calm and simple modern furniture that treads an attractive path between the monastically plain and the highly decorative—in other words it is eminently usable and fits as easily and beautifully into the country drawing room as the dockside loft. All the furniture is designed by the interior architect Henry Becq and is made mainly out of poplar or ash, which he either leaves natural or tints black or white. It's the place to go for clean-lined bookcases, elegant tables, simple and comfortable chairs and sofas, as well as a line of cream or white pottery, bowls and lamps, and some wonderfully comfortable and clean-lined leather chairs.

Blanc d'Ivoire, 104 rue du Bac, Paris 75007; +33 1 42 22 87 12. It's featured in every French design magazine and is chock full of Gallic charm—more *bastide* than *château*. Think Provence rather than the Loire. This is the place for romantic home furnishings in a modern mood—gauzy tablecloths and bedspreads made from hand-embroidered organdie, cream and beige quilted bedspreads, steel gray silk cushions, simple lamps of wood or metal, clean-lined bedside tables in ebonized wood, and a host of props that are easy enough to take home. Look for cushions in quilted cream or white as well as some gentle, faded florals and some quilts in velvet or satin that reflect the new glamour coming into the modish interior. It's the place, too, for subtly aged armoires, or handsome refectory tables. The props, in other words, for the life we wish we had.

Michèle Aragon, 21 rue Jacob, Paris 75006. Michèle Aragon's shop could come straight out of a classic old French movie. Here are all the ingredients for *la vie du château,* from antique red and white linen cloths, monogrammed sheets and tablecloths, sweetly floral quilts to old green majolica, crystal glasses, and anything else that a grand chatelaine might no longer have a need for. It's a wonderful place to rummage in and the stock is different every time you visit, but what is constant is the taste behind it all—the eye that loves the old, the finely worked, that goes for a certain sort of sophisticated rustic Gallic charm. Allow plenty of time to browse.

Also in the area and not to be missed: **Olario** at 30 rue Jacob, Paris 75006, for pretty French accessories including the wonderful delicate cream tableware made by Astier de Villatte. **Catherine Memmi** (very austere, impeccably refined and very expensive furniture, linens and a small range of clothing) at 32/34 rue Saint Sulpice, Paris 75006; +33 1 44 07 02 02, and Maison de Famille (huge glass lanterns, inexpensive glass, great welcoming dining tables, side tables and characterful lamps) at 29 rue Saint Sulpice, Paris 75006; +33 1 56 24 96 91. **Christian Liaigre**, 61 rue de Varenne, Paris 75007; +33 1 45 51 46 32, the undisputed leader of the minimalist set—lots of dark, streamlined furniture with not a decorative twirl in sight. **Julie Prisca**, at 46 rue du Bac, Paris 75007; +33 1 45 48 13 29, has bleached oak and ebonized tables, white linen-covered sofas, and lots of metalwork (chairs, mirrors, accessories) as well as lacquerware and a host of desirable small objects. Don't forget **Muriel Grateau**, 37 rue de Beaune, Paris 75007; +33 1 40 20 42 82. Design fundis around the world make little pilgrimages to Muriel Grateau where they find delicious ceramics, table linens, cutlery, glass and what she calls "the things that are personal and so close to the user—all the little things that finish off the look of an interior." Catherine Deneuve and Calvin Klein are both said to be fans. As a matter of interest she has also moved into jewelry now, which is fabulously strong and sculptural.

The Marais

Caravane, 6 rue Pavée, Paris 75004; +33 1 44 61 04 20. Founded by one of Paris's best-known interior stylists, Françoise Dorget, who used to be the stylistic spirit behind Etamine, the wallpaper and fabric house, Caravane offers a beguiling mix of things new and old—the sort of exotic collection a sophisticated, traveled voyager might collect. It has a big north-African (particularly Moroccan) influence tempered by a northern refinement—a sort of Ali-Baba-meets-loft-style living.

Villa Marais, 40 rue des Francs-Bourgeois, Paris 75003; +33 1 42 78 42 40. Very quirky indeed, with a mix of the contemporary (mostly of the kitsch variety) and the antique—it's called eclectic. Chandeliers vulgar enough to boggle the eye jostle side by side with delicate Fortuny lights; a wonderfully decorated old German antique chest sits beside a deep lacquered cupboard from China. It's a good place to browse for the strange, the unorthodox, the one-off present. Also in the area and not to be missed: Village Saint-Paul is much closer to the centre of Paris than the flea markets of Clignancourt and consists of a cluster of antique shops grouped in a haphazard way around the old streets and courtyards off the rue Saint-Paul and the rue Charlemagne. There are both inexpensive *brocantes* (the less expensive, junkier end of the market) and pukka *antiquaires* (expensive objects of some intrinsic worth), all of which provide inexpensive entertainment even if they don't always deliver up the unmissable bargain.

How to Do the Paris Puces

On Fridays the market is reserved for official dealers, and Saturdays and Sundays are for amateur trawlers like you and me. There's no need to get there too early. Dress for comfort, take cash if you can for the smaller things (though most stalls do take credit cards) and get on the Metro to Porte de Clignancourt. There are easily spotted kiosks where you can get maps of the market place. Give the cheap market stalls a miss and head straight for the rue des Rosiers.

The market you want first, if you're after charming pieces of furniture and accessories for the house and garden, is Marché Paul Bert and the things to look out for are wonderful old fireplaces, painted provincial furniture, old armoires, mirrors, chandeliers (there's something about French ones that gives a bit of oomph to almost any interior), bits and pieces of architectural salvage (particularly good for those with large gardens), old lights, and a hundred and one other things to perk up a room. If you're looking for a dining table, the Marché Paul Bert is a good place to find one of those charming old fruitwood farmhouse tables or something originally made for the garden or conservatory in wrought iron and marble.

The Marché Vernaison is filled with mostly rather smaller stands, all specializing in something, whether it be pictures, tapestries, faded toile de Jouy or military memorabilia. Linen fetishists should home in on Janine Giovannoni, Stand 141, at the corner of Allées 3 and 7, who has a cache of the sort of linen one wishes one's grandmother had kept. Serpette has biggish furniture, including a stand selling vast numbers of leather chairs.

A Few Good Web Sites

www.fabulousandfrench.co.uk offers all the main ingredients of the French provincial look.

www.hiddenart.com has lots of craft-made items—everything from glass to small tables, cushions, or bowls.

www.eurofurniture.com and **www.intirium.com** both sell good modern furniture at good prices.

Go to Marché Biron for good solid bourgeois furniture, if that's your taste—great big ornate sideboards and highly embellished chests, as well as tapestries that would suit an ancestral wall.

Scouring these three markets can be done in a day and all still seem to have plenty of those beguiling French pieces that are such an essential part of the boho or the pale French provincial look. Just don't be too disappointed by the prices—bargains are thin on the ground.

How do you get it all home? *Pas de problème.* Hedley's Humpers (+33 1 48 13 01 02; www.hedleyshumpers.com), right on the rue de Rosiers in the Marché Paul Bert, will ship it for you.

Have a steaming cup of coffee and a good croissant at the Petit Landais at 96 rue de Rosiers and a big bowl of mussels for lunch at Le Petit Navire, on the corner of the rue Paul Bert and rue de Rosiers.

But a word of warning: shopping in the Marché aux Puces is still fun, and you can still find charming decorative pieces, but cheap it isn't.

THE GREAT OUTDOORS

I'm no horticulturist. I've spent all my life living in cities and, if I'm not in a city, I try to go to wild, uncultivated wildernesses. Spending hours a week, let alone half a lifetime, in the cold, damp outdoors bent over flowerbeds, as serious garden lovers do, is not my idea of a good time. *But* we do have two tiny bits of outdoor space: a pocket handkerchief of a garden at the back of the house and a minute roof terrace high up at the back of the house.

They are both a lesson in how to conjure up a little bit of magic in a very small space. Stephen Woodhams, a well-known British garden designer, created both of them for me.

Personally, I think there are two approaches to having a small space and I've seen both work beautifully. One is to make it a wild, mad, overgrown plot, the walls suffused with climbing roses, clematis, jasmine, ivy, and any other plant you can force upwards and sideways. The ground is then covered with pots and urns, each sprouting its own glorious assortment of blooms, to create a wonderfully romantic, flower-filled garden. Add some rustic curvy wrought-iron furniture for eating out of doors, and you might feel as if you're in a country garden dell. I've known several hugely successful very small urban gardens that have brought off this look brilliantly.

The other approach—the one Stephen produced for us for our little patch—is more architectural and relies on some theatrical panache. Our back garden sports just four huge (and I mean *huge*) white flowerpots—they must be about six feet high and about three-and-a-half feet wide; we had to hire a crane to swing them over the roof. They give the garden a touch of magic that nothing small and pint-sized could ever have given it. (In white fiberglass, they cost about $700 apiece, plus delivery.) One has a giant yucca that we'd nurtured for years indoors and is now thriving outdoors. The other three, the ones visible from the kitchen window, each have a large bay tree in the center, which is underplanted according to the season: bulbs in winter to bring us pleasure in the spring, impatiens in one color (pure white one year, deep pink another) in the summer. If we wanted to be really trendy we could underplant with lettuces or cabbages—all tightly packed—as Stephen did for one of his exhibitions last year. The upkeep is minimal, which suits us just fine. He gave us lighting inset into the steps leading to the basement and in the pots themselves, so at night the uplighters illuminate the trees—magic. I found a beautifully sturdy and plain rectangular table and chairs that were very inexpensive and are a perfect soft greyish-greenish color that blends in beautifully with the soft grays of the English sky. And that's it.

Up on our tiny roof garden, Stephen's vision was to take what he (truthfully) called a "nothing area" and make it magical. He wanted to maximize the planting and yet take up minimal floor space. He had to be careful with the weight on the roof (we've "done" burst pipes; we don't want to "do" collapsed roofs), so he decided that one of the two huge planters that he planned would be made to measure to fill in a strange oblong gap along one side wall where a protrusion in the wall below could take most of the weight. The other planter was also made to measure to fit a space between the railing and the stairs and it, too, was to be bolted to the wall to take the weight off the roof.

The bigger of the two planters has something like a four-feet worth of planting, while the smaller has about two and a half feet. "Most people," says Stephen, "make the mistake of having planters that are too small and then they're surprised that their plants die. If you want big lush plants you need big lush planters." Ours are each nearly three feet deep, with one-third of the depth taken up with drainage (using clay granules) and two-thirds with lightweight compost.

The planters are painted battleship grey, which, according to Stephen, is a great background for plants and which gives the terrace a suitably urban, slightly hip, industrial feel. They're stuffed with plants, devised to give a mixture of seasonal effects, and they both look glorious already. Two of the climbers are evergreen (*Garrya elliptica* will have silvery grey catkins come the winter and it's next to a trachelospermum that has heavenly, sweet-scented flowers from May through to September). There are purple thistles, a vigorous *Solanum jasminoides* (that will give lots of white flowers from June until September), an olive tree, some wonderful silvery-grey grasses, a fantastic Chinese bamboo, and lots of other things with long botanical names. We both decided it would be nice to plant a clematis—one very pale blue, one deep burgundy—at the outer end of each planter so that they could, in time, cover the railings.

At the edge of the front of the terrace are three huge, oversized, cylindrical, lightweight, galvanized-steel containers topped with balls of boxwood topiary. As Stephen put it, "You need something over-scaled, architectural, gutsy, and sculptural—after all, you're in the middle of London, not suburbia." He was right. They're splendid.

Once again lighting makes the garden wonderful on a summer night. "You don't want floodlights," said Stephen, "just something gentle and magical." There's an extra plug so that you can read up there at night if you feel like it. The irrigation system is completely automatic and computerized so that we can go away for weeks (we should be so lucky) and not come back to horticultural devastation.

I dithered about the furniture, being temporarily beguiled by the Provençal charm of Grange's wrought-iron *lit de repos:* I had had visions of lounging about reading novels on it but it didn't suit the persona that the terrace had acquired, which needed something sleek and urban. So what we have now is a couple of black Verner Panton molded resin chairs and a small stool as a table—the space is *very* small.

Our terrace must be like thousands of others that lie at the back of urban terraced houses—at about twelve feet by eight feet it is probably smaller than most—but it has amazed me to discover that such a small patch can give so much joy. Even the vista from the stairs gives pleasure. On a summer evening we can sit up there, enjoying the cool breeze and the view of what Stephen Woodhams calls "the borrowed landscape" (all the other trees and gardens belonging to others). Remember this as you contemplate your own patch, no matter how small— something can be done, if imagination and energy are brought to bear upon the problem.

Some Favorite Addresses

The San Francisco Flower Mart (640 Brannan Street, San Francisco 94107; 415-781-8410; www.sfflmart.com) is a brilliant place to look for urns, pots, window boxes, and vases, at amazingly good prices and with lots of choice. Not to mention plants and flowers, of course.

Le Prince Jardinier, 37 rue de Valois, Paris 75001; +33 1 42 60 76 75, has some deliciously old-fashioned, traditional gardening implements, including watering cans, beautiful little tags for the garden, wonderful aprons and the like.

R. K. Alliston (www.rkalliston.com) has lovely classic planters, pots, string, pruning scissors, hand cream, candles, and all those traditional gardening things.

Marston & Langinger (192 Ebury Street, London SW1W 8UP; +44 20 7881 5730, and 117 Mercer St., New York

10012; 212-965-0434, and at www.marston-and-langinger
.com) is quite simply a delightful shop, filled with really pretty
charming things, not just for gardens but also for conservatories, patios, and roof terraces. There are lovely pressed-glass
plates and sundae dishes, as well as flowers and wrought-iron
planters. Also dramatic hurricane lamps and candle holders for
that indispensable aid to magic out of doors—candles.

Frances Hilary's Horticultural Gifts by Post (www
.franceshilary.com) sells hammocks, night lights, garden tubs,
and all the appurtenances the well-appointed garden needs.

www.springhillnursery.com delivers plants for pots, window boxes or indoors and has a huge variety at great prices.

www.henandhammock.co.uk is the Web site for those
who hate waste. It sells planters (actually rather wonderful)
made from recycled tires, glass lanterns made in Vietnam from
recycled glass, and teak furniture made from recycled teak, as
well as an extremely chic panama hat made, as all the best ones
are, in Ecuador.

The Conran Shop (www.conranusa.com) sells the world's
most delightful umbrella—a fantastically pretty green (or
cream) leafy, lacy parasol topped by a little bird—that is the
brainchild of that wonderful Dutch design collective called
Droog.

SIX

✻

food,
glorious
food

Eating Well

*Have the courage to serve the most homely dish
provided it is perfect of its kind.*
—Edouard de Pomiane

I see no point in eating bad food. It gives no pleasure, no proper nutrition and makes you fat. I love eating. I love wine. And real, proper food lies at the heart of one's domestic and social life. To sit at a table filled with friends and family, all enjoying the food I've provided and some decent wine, is one of life's great pleasures and—think about it—it doesn't, on the scale of things, cost a fortune.

Families that sit around tables enjoying Sunday lunches and evening suppers that have been properly (by which I don't mean elaborately) cooked and served tend to be closer and warmer than those who sit perched in front of the television set with fast food or takeout, not talking, not communicating. Families gathered around a table build up memories of intimacy and warmth that last throughout one's life. My children still remember the change in our eating habits when, after a small induction into the French way of life (via a holiday at the Club Méditerranée), I decided we, too, would eat with our children in the evening instead of giving them early supper and then having dinner by ourselves later. They remember that the food was revolutionized (for a few heady months we had a wonderful girl from Avignon doing the cooking) and the end of the day was transformed as they spent some real time with their parents. They have each decided in their turn to do it with their own children as soon as they are old enough. In many countries family life is disintegrating and families don't eat together as regularly as they once used to do. This seems to me deeply sad and something that over the years must wear away at the fabric of family life.

It's over dinner and lunch tables that all over the world we entertain our friends. By indulging in that age-old ritual of breaking bread together and drinking wine, we bond as families, as friends. So I have no truck with people who go to no trouble at all. I understand that we're busy and some of us are busier than others but it's never been easier to serve decent food with less trouble. I do know that cooking does take a certain amount of time. As a seriously distinguished writer Brenda Maddox put it to me one day, "The thing is that when you're cooking there are all sorts of other things you're *not* doing." In other words, it's not that cooking isn't pleasurable—it is, immensely—*but* if you've got a deadline to deliver, an operation to perform or a brief to master, you can't cook at the same time. *So* this chapter is not for those of you who are expert cooks and love nothing more than setting to in the kitchen. It's for those like me who love good food, don't want to eat junk and want to see their friends and families, but don't have the sort of time they'd like in which to do it all.

For just as the writer Shirley Conran always claimed that life was too short to stuff a mushroom, I think that life is too short to eat junk or to serve up lousy food. Anyway, these days there's no excuse. Peapod (www.peapod.com) is a wonder of the Western world. Dean & Deluca deserves a halo for the difference it's made to the working woman's life. Good meat and fish can be bought online. Farmers markets take fresh, gutsy and homemade food to almost every corner of the country, even to downtown Los Angeles, and bring to the experience of shopping in person something of the élan we all learned to admire in the French.

I grew up in South Africa at a time when food, in spite of the amazing quality of the natural ingredients, was mostly what you might call abysmal. It was Elizabeth David's sensuous prose that awoke in me a love of food, not to mention a deep desire to live in France. If you belong to the younger generation and haven't read her books, it's time you did. One heavenly summer in France my perception of food, of its cultural and geographical roots, of its life-giving daily pleasures, was awakened. We'd taken a villa in La Baule in Brittany, and with a three-year-old in one hand and a new baby in the other, and Elizabeth David's paperback *French Provincial Cooking* by my side, I embarked on a culinary educational journey.

As the children slept in the searing afternoon heat, I would read Elizabeth David under the shady trees. By the time they awoke I knew what I was going to cook and we'd head for the butcher, the fishmonger, the market. Every day I made a different dish. One day it was pork chops spiked with juniper berries baked in stock or white wine between layers of onions and potatoes. On another it was *paupiettes de veau* or a richly aromatic *boeuf en daube*. I learned that a simple omelette properly done, a green salad, some cheese and a piece of perfectly ripe fruit are better than many a formulaic fancy restaurant meal. Elizabeth David was also fanatical about eating seasonally. That way the food had real flavor, the fruit was properly ripe and nothing needed complicated treatment.

Some of that sounds a bit old-fashioned, now that so many of us have so little time, but though many of her dishes take a long time to cook they don't take much time to prepare. Take a classic braised rolled loin of veal. If you've bought it from a good butcher, all you need to do is to soften an onion, a carrot, some leeks, brown the veal all over, add white wine and herbs, toss it in a slow oven for two to three hours and there you have the basis of a delicious meal. I'm rather a fan of *petits pois* (and I even like the French canned or bottled *petits pois*) and will add them about ten minutes from the end to cook in the hot juices.

These days old-fashioned dishes are coming back. When Tom Parker Bowles (yes, that's Camilla's son) married Sara Buys, the wedding feast consisted of oysters and champagne to start with, his own fantastic recipe for cottage pie (the recipe is given on page 297) to follow, and a pudding (which is what is known in the United States as a dessert—i.e., something sweet and delicious) that I now cannot remember. I just know it was fabulous, so much more satisfying than itsy-bitsy fancy things of heaven-knows-what.

Fish pies, lasagnas, *moussakas,* risottos, and roast chicken: all these are heart-warming dishes that, if carefully made from fine ingredients (a chicken that has lived a decent life, been able to run around and has not been fed on its relations, for instance), are perennially comforting. You can always jazz them up a bit for guests: add shellfish or salmon to the fish pie, plus some cream and dill to its sauce; add truffles or porcini to the risotto; tuck some tarragon into the chicken, swirl some white wine around the roasting juices and add some crème fraîche to make a sauce.

Accompany these with crisp fresh mixed salad greens drizzled with a good virgin olive oil, a dash of balsamic vinegar and some herbs, and you can just follow up with cheese and fruit while leaving your guests feeling well looked after.

These days, though, you can get away without cooking if you know how to shop (I'm not addressing here that ever-increasing crowd who call in the caterers: lovely if you can afford it but most of us can't). It's all about sourcing. You need to track down the freshest of herbs if you don't grow your own (herbs do wonders for any dish), and know where to get the organic salmon, the fresh crab, the interesting cheese, the proper ceps and porcini, the fine virgin olive oil, the walnut oil, and great bread. You need to cook seasonally when flavors are at their freshest and most intense. There are also plenty of suppliers who can now be sourced online and will deliver. Some of the addresses can be found at the end of this chapter.

I've had some of the best meals of my life in the houses of friends who don't really cook but take trouble over sourcing the very best. One friend dishes up wonderful food in her country house and not until the weekend is over do you realize that very little cooking has gone on. Saturday lunch is usually a vast dish of fresh crab, bought (ready cooked) first thing in the morning from a fishmonger right by the sea. It's served with a dish of garlicky mayonnaise, a huge bowl of green leaves, some sliced tomatoes with basil, and new potatoes, all from the garden, scattered with herbs.

Sunday lunch is a socking great sirloin or fillet of beef cooked to perfection (all crispy on the outside, rosy pink on the inside) by the husband on the grill outside. It comes with baby carrots still with their tops on, tiny peas and more new potatoes. It's followed by great cheese and strawberries from the garden dipped in balsamic vinegar in the summer or something like poached pears in winter. All accompanied by delicious wines. Not cheap, I know, but it does save the cook getting frazzled.

Another friend, the writer and journalist Victoria Mather, always serves up heavenly food but it is simple in the extreme. It could be quails eggs to start with, asparagus in season or smoked salmon, or a big plate of lovely charcuterie. She'll follow it with a fillet of beef ("I only ever cook it for twenty minutes") and prefers salads to vegetables ("Saves that last-minute frazzle and getting your face all red"), though she will do new potatoes. She's lucky in that she has a really good butcher nearby but she gets her vegetables (seasonal, of course) from the greenmarket.

For an after-theatre supper when it all has to be ready in a flash, she'll do a Spanish tortilla (eggs with potato and onion) or scrambled eggs and smoked salmon topped with red caviar (but she serves the scrambled eggs cold) and follows it up with a *tarte tatin* from a good patisserie. Really good bangers and mash are another favorite—but the bangers come from a farmers market or a really good butcher, and the potatoes are put through a ricer. She, like me, is a fan of A. N. Wilson's fantastic way with shoulder of lamb, a really comforting winter dish. He puts the meat into a good ovenproof dish, covers it with two large cans of haricot beans and their liquid, two chopped onions, ten shallots, six tomatoes, some tomato purée and two glasses of white wine. He tucks in some bay leaves and rosemary, and then puts it in a low oven for four (yes, four) hours. It goes down as a particular treat with children. But do take care to cut away as much fat as you can before you cook it, as otherwise it can tend to be a little on the greasy side.

☞ *If you're going to keep it simple, then you must be wildly, madly generous. Great platters of fresh foods—good cheeses, salads, chunky slices of rare beef, fat pink shrimp, charcuterie—look wonderfully welcoming and hospitable.*

Presentation is also vitally important. Herbs sprinkled over things can do wonders—for the look as well as the taste. Use attractive dishes and make the food look fantastic. You should aim for only the best and freshest of ingredients. Smoked salmon, for instance, is still a delicious treat but only if it is the best—that nasty, pink, oily farmed stuff isn't worth eating, in my view. And it should be offered with really good bread, now available almost everywhere. Buy the smoked salmon from somewhere like Pacific Northwest Best Fish Co. (www.pacific nwbest.com), where the fish is organically farmed (in wide-open tidal pens) and they smoke it themselves. Chicken should be organic and free-range, it goes without saying. Get your beef, pork, bacon and their like from the best sources (the addresses are on pages 298–299) and there are now growing numbers of dedicated farmers who farm named breeds in humane ways without pesticides or chemicals.

When it comes to wanting to feed our friends, our wise mentor Edouard de Pomiane believed that "For a successful dinner there should never be more than eight people. One should prepare *only one good dish*." In other words, for the other two courses (usually, presumably, the starter and the third course) *faites simple* (by which you will have gathered by now that I do not mean slapdash). Now that we have good *traiteurs,* delicatessens and patisseries, you can easily top and tail the meal with something bought. There's also no need any more to stick to the structure of the three-course meal. I sometimes like doing something more Middle Eastern and have lots of dips (most delicatessens do very good hummus, eggplant purées and *tzatziki*) and grilled vegetables (eggplant, red peppers, roasted onions), which can also be found in good delicatessens, followed by something simple and grilled, like crispy chicken dressed with herbs and lemon juice.

I also sometimes do a great big tureen of aromatic fish soup, dead easy to do. Then I jazz up some fresh mayonnaise with chili and garlic to serve as a sort of *rouille,* offer an herby green salad and gorgeous bread, followed by cheese and fruit, and it always goes down with a wow. If I'm really, really pushed for time and need to produce a supper for sixteen—or even a smarter dinner for six—I've learned ways to doll up the best supermarket food. It may not be up to the finest homemade but it's better than not seeing your friends or making excuses not to welcome visitors. For a buffet supper for sixteen when I had endless deadlines on the go, I've taken packets of mushroom risotto, decanted them into a vast baking dish (which makes it look homemade) and heated them up in the oven, remembering to double or triple the heating times. I've then sautéed some wild mushrooms (I always keep packs of dried porcini on hand) in a mix of butter and oil, which I stirred in, adding a tiny bit of truffle oil and showered it with chopped parsley, and then served it with bowls of freshly grated Parmesan. At least three people asked me for the recipe.

I mostly avoid pasta, not because I don't like it (I *love* it) but because it's fattening (all those carbs). If that doesn't worry you, you can whip up endlessly delicious fast-food dishes using fresh pasta (it takes only three minutes to cook) and many of the bottled sauces you can buy are terrific. I first came across fresh pesto when it was served to us by Italian friends in a beach hut near San Remo—mixed in with fresh spaghetti and proper Parmesan, it was a revelation. But to my mind the best pasta dish of all is the *tagliarini al bosco* from the River Café's first cookbook. It's a creamy herby asparagus pasta dish that is probably my husband's favorite dish in the world (though not especially fast, it's not difficult).

Most supermarkets these days sell excellent ranges of good ready-prepared food (no E numbers, stabilizers, preservatives, artificial colors, flavorings, or sweeteners) that require very little effort at home—look for chicken and prosciutto parcels, all nicely skewered with a sprig of rosemary, or a pretty decent beef Wellington or a nice big piece of salmon with chopped spring onion, red pepper and a soy sauce topping. Add a green salad, or a green vegetable, and either new potatoes or mashed. I'm addicted to mashing potatoes with olive oil—it's better for the arteries and I prefer the taste.

If you're really, really stuck on a dank Sunday evening (as once happened to me when some friends I'd forgotten I'd asked called at about four P.M. just as we were plunked out on the

sofa after rather too enjoyable a lunch to say they were going to
be a little late for dinner), you'll have to turn to the pantry.
Keep certain things always in store: tins of tomatoes; Carnaroli
rice for risottos; good chicken and fish stock in the freezer,
proper yellow-fin tuna preserved in oil in bottles; dried mushrooms; olives; ceps; some good tapenade.

Dean & Deluca has a brilliant selection of beautiful
ingredients—such as truffles, balsamic jelly, and sauces. Now
that you can access them online (www.deandeluca.com), and
they'll deliver, they're well worth keeping in the pantry. Have
really good ice cream in the freezer: Blue Bell, Ben & Jerry's,
Mayfield, or United Dairy Farmers to name just a few.

It's worth trying out a few local takeout services to see if
anybody does it well. New Yorkers can be rescued by Zabar's
(245 West Eightieth Street, New York 10024; 212-787-2000;
www.zabars.com), which will deliver freshly prepared meals,
such as a ready-roasted organic chicken or poached salmon,
and sides. Gordon Ramsay it isn't but it's fresh, healthy, and
very nice, thank you, when you're in a jam.

☞ *If you're going to dish up takeout (and provided you choose good ones
and serve them so that they look good, why on earth not? My mantra, as you
may already have gathered, being that it's better to compromise than not to see
your friends because you can't find the time to do it all perfectly), there are three
golden rules: keep the lighting glamorously low (candles, candles, candles); hide
the evidence (bags, boxes); and garnish, garnish, garnish.*

You can finish with one great gorgeous cheese (*not* a dinky
little selection with assorted cheese biscuits, please), like a huge
mound of sharp cheddar; a great big camembert, unpasteurized
for the best flavor (try wrapping it in puff pastry and baking it
at 425° F for twenty minutes and serving with a frisée salad); or
one of the heavenly American cheeses now being made; a generous wedge of fresh Parmesan; a great big stilton at Christmas or a

Stinking Bishop if you can get your hands on it, which you dip into with spoons and serve with a crisp green salad. They are all so much more appealing than teeny-weeny bits and pieces. Charles Martell makes Stinking Bishop on his farm near Dymock in Gloucestershire (+44 1531 890 637), though since it featured in the recent Wallace & Gromit movie he has been flooded with orders. Alternatively, it's hard to beat a perfectly ripe pear and a piece of Taleggio as a fine way to end a meal.

For pudding, most city dwellers live near a good patisserie these days, but even supermarkets are offering up really good puddings. You have to wend your way carefully through the ready-made section but if you can find it, a good, admirably sharp *tarte au citron* is a nice accompaniment in the summer to lots of berries. Individual open apple tarts, straight from the bakery on the premises, are always terrific. Many fine grocers have now started selling cold individual lemon soufflés and créme brûlées in white porcelain pots, which means they can be transported straight from fridge to table. There are now delicious selections of chocolate "puds" (very seductive), which come in pretty little pots that you could produce in any company, as well as pots of lemon curd, which I serve with raspberries when in season. Delicious fruity puddings, once again in perfectly attractive plain white china dishes, go down a bundle. Even simpler still, Greek yogurt topped with honey and toasted almonds or walnuts takes some beating.

Don't forget—as if you could—Whole Foods—there are several dotted around the country (check the addresses on their Web site, www.wholefoods.com), and they are a wonder to behold. Never will you have seen so many varieties of shrimp, bean, bread, cheese or anything else. They pride themselves on quality and abundance. Go, look and wonder.

Nigel Slater's *Real Fast Food* is a classic for those who want proper fast food, what he calls "fresh food, bright flavors and relaxed eating." None of the dishes takes more than thirty minutes to cook and most are exactly the sort of fresh, robust modern food that most of us want to eat today. Here, though, I'm parting with some of my own favorite quick dishes. Some are really obvious but it's useful sometimes to be reminded of them. All of these I produce quite often and I hope they'll give you some ideas.

That said, I do think that being better organized would mean one could do all those long, slow-cooked dishes that Elizabeth David wrote about so evocatively. They often take very little time to prepare and are less likely to frazzle the nerves since they need less precision in their cooking times and usually no last-minute attention. You just need to put them in the oven ahead of time (which may sometimes mean cooking the previous night so that you can just reheat the following evening) and then let them simmer away, slowly allowing the flavors to mingle and work their magic.

TEN DEAD EASY STARTERS

1. **Melon soup.** Whiz together one large ripe orange-fleshed melon, half a cucumber, 2 teaspoons of red-wine vinegar, and some salt and pepper. Slowly add some olive oil to the mixture to emulsify. Chill and serve.

2. **Chilled green-pea soup.** Soften a chopped onion in a little oil, add one pound of peas (fresh or frozen), some fresh mint and twenty fluid ounces of chicken stock. Cook for five minutes. Add salt and pepper, and purée. Serve cold with a little crème fraîche stirred into it and some chopped chives.

3. **A great platter** overflowing with the freshest of shrimp from a fishmonger (or, better still, if you've time, cook your

own in a big pan with some ginger and garlic) and a huge bowl of mayonnaise—homemade if you have time, otherwise buy it from stores or delicatessens. Serve with fresh crusty bread and some farmhouse butter.

4. **Prosciutto di parma** or, better still, Prosciutto di San Daniele or the Spanish *pata negra* ham (if you can find it; try www.tienda.com), curled over roasted red onions on a bed of rocket. Sprinkle with toasted pine nuts and drizzle with olive oil. Or air-cured ham and fresh figs (after washing the figs, open them up into quarters). Or Bresaola with proper buffalo mozzarella from a good delicatessen, a base of arugula, a trickle of the best olive oil and shards of fresh Parmesan.

5. **Fig and mozzarella salad.** In the summer months, make a base of peppery arugula and on top put a combination of ripe figs, quartered, ripe nectarines and chunks of proper buffalo mozzarella. Swirl over good olive oil and some balsamic vinegar.

6. **Asparagus.** You can serve it lots of ways. Either simply hot (with melted butter and Parmesan cheese or hollandaise sauce) or cold (with a French vinaigrette). Or wrap it in prosciutto and grill until browned.

7. **Jellied consommé**, good canned (it must be from the fridge so that it is properly jellied; Campbell's is the best brand, I've found). Serve with sour cream and the cheapskate's caviar (black fish roe eggs), topped with chopped chives.

8. **Potted shrimp.** A great English classic, potted shrimp is fundamentally nothing more than little brown shrimp in a tiny china pot conserved with a topping of melted butter, which then solidifies in the fridge. Serve with brown bread and lemons.

9. **Beet salad.** Juliennes (this is important: don't on any account cut them into rounds, which reminds me of school and desperate bleeding salads) of beet (*not* the ones doused

in vinegar; freshly cooked versions are now available in supermarkets if you don't have time to cook your own), mixed with crumbled Roquefort cheese and topped with walnut pieces. Combine with a walnut oil dressing and lots of parsley. Serve on a base of arugula.

10. **Chicken liver salad.** Toss some chicken livers in butter until crisp outside but still a bit pink inside. Slide onto a mixture of arugula rocket, crisp torn romaine and other green leaves. Deglaze the pan with some vinegar, scrape up all the juicy bits and pour over the leaves. This works nicely with lardons as well.

Ten Easy Main Courses

1. **Roast chicken.** It must be free-range organic (buy it from www.sheepdrove.com). Stuff it with a lemon cut in half and masses of tarragon, dribble over olive oil and roast. When cooked, lift out, add white wine to the juices, swirl in cream and it makes a heavenly sauce. If you want to upgrade the meal do the same thing with guinea fowl (from Whole Foods). Serve with a crisp green salad and new potatoes.

2. **Roast fillet of beef** (or grouse or pheasant in season). Timing is all. Brown it all over so you get a crispy outside and then roast at a high temperature (400° F) for ten minutes per one pound. Serve in chunky slices with crème fraîche spiked with fresh horseradish or lots of mustard, herby new potatoes and a green salad. I also like to serve it accompanied by little branches of slow-roasted small tomatoes on the vine (but you need a separate oven to do that).

3. **Pork fillet.** Cut into rounds, fry until brown on either side and cooked through. Swirl a little white wine in the juices, add cream and dash of mustard. Serve with noodles or mashed potato. If you have time, mushrooms make a nice addition to the sauce.

4. **Scallops.** Fry some bacon in a sturdy frying pan. Add fresh scallops (dry them on paper towels first) until crisp on one side, then turn over to cook the other side. Add some shrimp, a little white wine (it must bubble), some cream and lots of herbs. This takes no more than five or six minutes. Serve either on a mound of rice, or a bed of watercress, mâche, and arugula. Or serve on a bed of puréed green peas.

5. **Rack of lamb.** Rub with olive oil and rosemary and roast for twenty-five minutes in a hot oven (400° F) over a bed of halved onions, bottled artichoke hearts and parboiled halved potatoes. This is fabulously easy. Sprinkle with loads of parsley and other herbs.

6. **Steak.** Buy the best filet mignon. Sear in a mixture of olive oil and butter. How long depends upon how rare you like them. When done, remove from the pan, add some red wine (let it bubble), lots of mustard and crème fraîche. You can make it more elaborate by cooking a little onion and some mushrooms in some butter first. Remove from the pan and add to the sauce when the steaks are cooked. Serve with heaps of mashed potato (I like it with olive oil but you may prefer butter) and a green salad.

7. **Fish.** This is tricky to time but if you're just a small group (no more than four), trout with almonds is dead simple. Dip the trout in flour, and then fry in a mixture of butter and oil. When it has crisped on the outside and just turned opaque on the inside, remove it from the pan, deglaze with some white wine, add a little more butter and some blanched almonds, and cook until brown. Pour the juices over the trout, add lots of lemon juice and parsley and serve with whatever you like (new potatoes and baby green peas or beans are lovely). Alternatively, go for a whole fish (sea bass is prohibitively expensive, but you can doll up a fresh side of haddock with herbs and lemon juice), which you simply sprinkle with olive oil, add fennel and fresh dill, and then bake—but you must check your timings so that you don't overcook it.

8. **Cod**. You can bake cod (fry it skin-side down first to give it a crisp surface, then bake until cooked), serve it on a bed of lentils (which makes a change from potatoes) and give it a lift with a salsa verde sauce. (To make the sauce, whiz in a blender a mass of parsley, mint, basil, some capers and cornichons [or gherkins], anchovies if you like them, and olive oil until you have a lumpy, emulsified sauce.)

9. **Pork chops**. If you get these from a reputable butcher, they make great quick easy food (from a supermarket they tend to be tough). Simply brown them on either side in a small amount of hot oil and butter. When brown add one whole head of endives, halved, per chop. Brown the endives on both sides. Then season, add a glass of white wine, cover and fry gently until cooked—about fifteen minutes. Remove from the pan when done. Stir a little more butter into the juices and pour over the chops. Serve with new potatoes or noodles and a salad. This can also be done with chicken pieces.

10. **Salmon**. You can do lots of things with small salmon steaks. Simply fry them crisply in a combination of butter and oil (the oil helps stop the butter burning), and when they are done, deglaze the pan with some white wine, adding lots of dill, lemon juice and some crème fraîche. Alternatively, try something more Eastern and bake with a topping of chopped spring onions and finely chopped chili, ginger, and garlic. When done, serve with a sauce made quickly from more chopped ginger, honey and soy sauce all mixed together. Serve with green vegetables, new potatoes, and a salad.

Ten Easy "Puds"

1. **A simple bowl of mixed berries** with crème fraîche or try strawberries in balsamic vinegar. If you have time (it needs to drain for a few hours or, better still, overnight), make *coeurs à la crème* as an accompaniment. Line heart-shaped

white china moulds that have holes in the bottom with muslin and put in a mixture (all whipped together) of cream, yogurt and some unsalted cream cheese, chill and allow to drain. When firm, turn out the little heart-shaped mounds. Lovely with crunchy sugar. If you're short of time, serve with *fromage blanc*.

2. **Stuffed peaches.** Crush *amaretti* and stuff into the hollow of stoned, halved peaches, spoon over some honey and grill, or put in a low oven for twenty minutes. Serve with chilled cream.

3. **Coffee delight.** Make a pint of strong, fabulous real coffee. When hot, add one packet of gelatin and stir until it's dissolved. Pour into a glass bowl to set. When firm, cover it first with a layer of whipped cream (or a mixture of yogurt and cream, or just crème fraîche) and crumble lots of *amaretti* over the top.

4. **Fruit and cheese.** One summer in the Dordogne, when on vacation with friends, after the children were all safely in bed, our nightly treat was a perfect peach, some sharp unsalted creamy cheese (Petit Suisse will also do nicely) and a glass of Monbazillac. I still think there's nothing more delicious though these days I'd take a bit more care over the quality of the dessert wine.

5. **Boodles Orange Fool** is dead easy. Soak a plain sponge cake (with no cream or jam in the middle) in *fresh* orange or grapefruit juice (both can be bought in a supermarket) and, when the juice is absorbed, mix in some whipped cream.

6. **Cold orange soufflé.** Elizabeth David's wonderful recipe from *A Book of Mediterranean Food*. Soak a half ounce of gelatin in one pint of fresh orange juice. Add two tablespoons of sugar. Heat and when nearly boiling pour over two well-beaten egg yolks. Combine thoroughly. When cool, mix in the stiffly beaten whites of the two eggs. Chill.

7. **Pears baked in wine.** Peel but leave the stalks on. Add three ounces of sugar per pound of pears and either sweet white

wine or red wine, mixed with water. Cook slowly in a low oven (200 to 300° F); one hour is enough if they're ripe, or up to three hours if they're hard.

8. **Poached fruit in Muscat.** Quinces are the most delicious but are hard to come by. Otherwise peaches are delectable, too, but are more delicate and need a shorter cooking time. Whenever I see quinces in the shops I grab them because they aren't easy to get hold of. I peel and cut them into thick slices and cook them very, very slowly in a low oven (something like two to two and a half hours) in Muscat or Sauterne, with a little added sugar and some spices to cut the sweetness—cinnamon, bay leaves, cloves, and cardamom. Dissolve the sugar, bring the wine to the boil, then put in the fruit. Serve when cool. Ambrosia.

9. **Baked bananas.** Cut them in half. Add some butter, brown sugar, orange or lemon juice, nutmeg, cinnamon and some honey. Bake for thirty minutes.

10. **Ice cream.** Most supermarkets have a good range made from proper ingredients like cream and eggs. You can add all sorts of toppings, ginger in syrup is my favorite, but defrosted berries, honey and chopped walnuts, crushed meringues and melted chocolate all work well.

A Word About Chocolate

We're trained from girlhood to think it's *not* allowed. Not everyone knows this but pure cocoa has no cholesterol-raising ingredients at all. Real chocolate is low in sugar and has lots of vitamins, while cocoa butter lowers blood cholesterol levels. And there's more good news: really good chocolate increases the levels of serotonin in the brain (serotonin is what makes us feel happy) and it also contains phenylethylamine, which is very similar to the chemicals released in our bodies when we fall in love. There—chocolate's allowed after all, and doesn't that feel better?

So on a cold winter's night you can now go for a guilt-free cup of heavenly hot chocolate. **Pierre Marcolini** at 485 Park Avenue, New York 10022 (212-755-5150 and at www.marcolini chocolatier.com) sells flakes of the purest 100 percent dark chocolate. Stir slowly into heated milk (skimmed to keep it guilt-free) and never let it boil. This is as different from the sugary, saturated-fat-infused commercial versions as Château Lafite is from supermarket *vino* and it comes in very chic black tins.

Demand for high-end chocolates is rising and in New York alone something like twelve new specialist chocolatiers have opened up shop in the last few years—all of them selling what are fashionably called "artisanal" (handmade to you and me) chocolates, all of them offering innovative, highly-specialized products and some of them introducing creative new ideas such as chocolate tastings, educational courses and special chocolate bars. Two of the best are **MarieBelle** at 484 Broome Street, New York 10013; 212-925-6999 (fabulous retro packaging and a heavenly chocolate drink that comes laced with chili), and **Kee's Chocolates**, 80 Thompson Street, New York 10012; 212-334-3284, where you can see the chocolates being made by hand.

The classic French chocolatier **La Maison du Chocolat** has two shops in Manhattan—in Rockefeller Center (no. 30; 212-265-9404) and at 1018 Madison Avenue, New York 10075; 212-744-7117 (find them online at www.lamaisonduchocolat .com).

SOME IDEAS ON DRINKS

I'm not going to embark on a discourse about wine here, largely because I'm not an expert (I tend to buy quite a lot from an online wine merchant—www.wine.com is quite popular—I just click the mouse and the wine arrives, is usually terrific and some time later I notice the bank account is down rather more than I'd remembered) and partly because all newspapers dispense good advice regularly. However, I do wish more people would go to a bit more trouble over nonalcoholic alternatives. I love wine but can't drink too much of it without getting a hangover. Here are a few nonalcoholic suggestions:

The best tomato juice is made from puréed and sieved fresh sweet tomatoes, seasoned and spiced. I first tasted it in Spain and thought I'd gone to heaven. I assume they peeled and deseeded the tomatoes first.

Funkin Purées are made from fresh white peaches, strawberries, passion fruit and raspberries, and they make brilliant smoothies, can be poured over ice cream or can make instant Bellinis (add the peach to your favorite champagne or prosecco). They come in very groovy packaging and are $8.99 a pack from liquor stores or online at www.wallywine.com.

Ripe puréed melons make a deliciously refreshing drink that can be lightened with a little iced soda water and zipped up with some fresh ginger or mint.

Dry Soda (888-379-7632 and at www.drysoda.com) makes all-natural plant-based sodas: kumquat, lavender, lemongrass, and rhubarb.

GUS (212-355-7454 and at www.drinkgus.com) does additive- and preservative-free lemon, ginger, pomegranate, and grape sodas.

Farmers' Markets

There are over four thousand farmers' markets in the country today. If you haven't already discovered them, the easiest way to do so is to tap into www.farmersmarketsusa.org and you'll be able to track down the one closest to where you live. Authentic farmers' markets consist of small stallholders, each of whom sells only things he or she has grown or raised personally. Many of them have expanded into producing dishes—soups, cakes, pies and the like, all of which have to be homemade, and while the ingredients are nearly always (one assumes) authentic, the quality of the finished product is variable. Trial and error at your local market will lead you to the suppliers whose wares you like. But some of the breads, homemade cheeses, cakes, soups and pâtés are truly delicious.

Some Good Greenmarkets

Berkeley Farmers' Markets, Berkeley, California; 510-548-3333. Tuesdays at Derby St.; Thursdays at Shattuck Ave.; and Saturdays at Center Street.

Dane County Farmers' Market, Capitol Square, Madison, Wisconsin; 608-455-1999. Wednesdays in the summer and Saturdays year-round.

Ferry Plaza Farmers' Market, Ferry Building, San Francisco, California; 415-291-3276. Tuesdays and Sundays until two.

Green City Market, Chicago, Illinois; 773-435-0280. Wednesdays and Saturdays in the summer.

The Los Angeles Farmers' Market, Los Angeles, California; 866-993-9211. Opens every day at nine A.M.

Pike Place Market, Seattle, Washington; 206-682-7453. Open seven days a week; closed on Thanksgiving, Christmas Day, and New Year's Day.

Portland Farmers' Market, Portland, Oregon; 503-241-0032. Wednesdays at Shemanski Park; Thursdays at Ecotrust and Eastbank; and Saturdays at Portland State University.

Union Square Greenmarket, New York, New York; 212-788-7476. Mondays, Wednesdays, Fridays, and Saturdays.

Tom Parker Bowles's Chili Cottage Pie

Serves 4

3 tablespoons olive oil

3 Thai chilies, finely chopped
  (deseeded and deveined for less heat)

2 medium red onions, coarsely chopped

1 pound organic ground beef

1 teaspoon tomato purée

1 can beef and sherry consommé

3 tablespoons Worcestershire sauce

a few shakes Tabasco

4 medium-size baking potatoes

generous lump of unsalted butter

splash of milk

freshly ground black pepper and salt

Heat the olive oil and sweat the chilies to infuse in the oil for 2 to 3 minutes. Add the onions and cook over a low heat until soft and brown (about 5 minutes). Turn up the heat a little and add the ground beef in handfuls, stirring into the onion. When all the onion and beef is mixed together and browned, add the tomato purée and stir to combine. After 1 minute, pour in the broth and sherry. Add the Worcestershire sauce and Tabasco, and stir again. Turn the heat down to a simmer and reduce for about 30 minutes. Keep tasting. In the meantime, peel the potatoes and throw into a large pan of cold, salted water. Bring to the boil and simmer until soft. Drain and put back into the pan over the heat (to dry off any excess water). Add the butter, a splash of milk, and mash. Turn the beef mixture into a shallow, oven-proof baking dish and cover with the potato. Dot the potato with chunks of butter, season with salt and pepper, and bake in a preheated oven (at 375° F) for 25 minutes. Serve with peas or lima beans, drenched in butter.

Markets Around the World

Even if you're not planning on doing any cooking, it's well worth browsing the best food markets. You can always come back with some cheese, sausages, or ceps. These are my favorites:

ENGLAND

Daylesford Organic in Daylesford, Gloucestershire, sells perfectly hung and butchered organically raised meat, homemade cheeses, dairy products, fruit and vegetables as well as a delicious selection of homemade breads, cakes, biscuits, soups, and other dishes.

In London, there is **Borough Market** down by London Bridge, which has transformed shopping for serious foodies, but there are many, many other farmers' markets dotted all over London from Blackheath to Ealing.

PICNICS

No climate in the world is less propitious to picnics than the climate of England, yet with a reckless-ness which is almost sublime, the English rush out of doors to eat a meal on every possible and impossible occasion.

—GEORGINA BATTISCOMBE IN *ENGLISH PICNICS*

I love picnics but there are, of course, picnics and picnics. There are the ones on top of a snowy mountain in the middle of a hundred square miles of wilderness (yes, really, when heli-skiing in British Columbia) when the hot soup and even hotter

PARIS

Marché Richard-Lenoir, just by the Place de la Bastille, is one the liveliest markets in Paris, and it's open on a Sunday. There's always a great selection of mushrooms.

Rue Cler in the 7th arrondissement has a wonderful village-y atmosphere, where French housewives often shop for Sunday lunch on their way home from church.

Rue Mouffetard in the 5th arrondissement is another charming little market for those who live in the neighborhood.

For picnics you can, of course, patronize **Fauchon** and **Hediard**, the twin grand food stores, but for a luxe picnic on the hoof, I think you couldn't do better than Flo Prestige, 42 Place du Marché Saint-Honoré. Here you can pick up charcuterie, foie gras, breads (in small portions or large), cheeses, *une douceur* for afterwards, wine, and anything else you might need.

chili con carne, served out of huge thermoses, were just perfect. There are the ones huddled by dunes, sheltering from the wind in what passes for a British summer, when some hot soup was what one longed for and humdrum sandwiches were what one got. There are rustic ones in France (our son has a house in the Cévennes, surrounded by woods and hills, and picnics are a big feature of time spent there) when one understands why La France Profonde is such a beguiling place—the fresh baguettes, the cheeses, tomatoes, olives, farm-made pâtés, good charcuterie, ripe peaches and grapes, and wine are better than anybody could wish for.

For country outings (point-to-points and country fairs, not to mention visits to the seaside), sturdier food is needed. A game or chicken pie, if one can find a good local supplier, is perfect, and drinks like homemade ginger beer and lemonade are ideal. It's great to end with some sharp cheese and fruit. For wintry picnics, hot soups are wonderfully restorative and things like stews and goulashes can be kept beautifully hot in a thermos. I'm not a sandwich fan—for me they're dull and never hit the spot.

And now, since we have finally got to the top of the Glyndebourne list and so can get tickets to its wonderful operas and we love Grange Park and Garsington opera almost as much, we indulge in grander picnics where a little more effort is needed.

Here is what I've learned about picnics. Without staff, bringing the fantasy of the perfect picnic to life is too burdensome even to try. When you read the details of the grand picnics that feature in novels or old-fashioned memoirs, there are always hordes of staff, huge joints of beef, elaborate mousses and a host of fancy dishes. The grand picnic that one conjures up in one's imagination would involve wicker baskets (a devil to carry), a beautiful linen cloth, a fine rug (even a faded Persian?), flickering candles, china, crystal, and wonderful food and drink, but all this involves much carrying to and fro, which becomes tiresome if the car isn't close to the picnic site—which in one sense defeats the point of the truly rustic picnic, which is to be far from roads and cars. If you happen to have a country house, on a summer evening you could replicate something like this at the end of your very own garden—a magical thing to do and not impossible without staff.

Otherwise I tone down my expectations. For opera festivals if the parking lot isn't too far from the picnic grounds, I have a routine that involves a folding table and chairs that fit in the trunk, an antique French linen cloth and linen napkins (extravagant, as we always get red wine on them, but worth it), and proper china and glass, but for any other sort of picnic I adopt a much more casual approach. I don't take a table and chairs but instead we sit on a waterproof rug with handles (from R. K. Alliston, www.rkalliston.com). I also love those traditional old plaid Welsh blankets called Carthenni, which have a bit of history attached to them but otherwise classic tartan blankets are pleasing to sit on and to look at. Then there's the cooler for the drinks. We start with champagne and move on to whatever wines my husband has chosen (though not too much because everybody has to drive home again afterwards).

In France, where long walks nearly always precede the picnic, all the children (even the four-year-olds) have light inexpensive picnic backpacks that include little plates, knives, forks and glasses, so that they can carry their own stuff while the adults haul the heavier things.

I have in my time done more elaborate picnics—strips of chicken marinated and then grilled, things wrapped in pastry, multi-layered confections of eggs and vegetables—but these days I find simpler food works best. I keep away from anything that could melt (obviously) or anything with a runny sauce, but on a really hot day I do like cold soups (a thermos keeps them cold very efficiently) and hot ones on cold days.

So here are some of the foods that have worked for us when we're in more elaborate mode.

Chilled pea or watercress soup or vichyssoise from a thermos are very summery. Smoked trout or smoked eel with some horseradish sauce and lemon juice, and thinly sliced buttered brown bread. A selection of crudités with dips from the supermarket (hummus, *tzatziki*, aubergine purée), though I decant them into little china pots to make them look prettier. Asparagus with vinaigrette and some shards of Parmesan, packed separately. Prosciutto di parma and figs (easier to cope with—and in my view nicer—than dealing with cutting up a melon and its seeds). Freshly cooked shrimp and some mayonnaise.

Cold fillet of beef—all crusty on the outside and pink on the inside, cut into nice thick slices and served with a creamy horseradish sauce.

Cold chicken, but only if organic and cooked the same morning with heaps of tarragon. Bought ready-cooked and cold from a supermarket is, in my view, a waste of money.

Cold pink rack of lamb—ideally cooked the same morning—with mint jelly or a spicy chutney is perfect.

Salmon is somehow more predictable so I don't do it but most people love it. Salmon trout is more delicate and good served with an herby, green mayonnaise.

With the above I serve new potatoes, cooked and tossed while still warm in a vinaigrette with lots of herbs, chopped scallions and chives, plus some baby tomatoes spiked with basil. Sometimes I vary the salads with a combination of peas, fava beans and feta cheese, or a combination of peas and snow peas, or green beans perked up with toasted almonds and some small chopped tomatoes.

Afterwards we have a great big slab of cheese and some crackers (taking bread, a bread knife, and butter is a complication too far), followed by fresh berries of some kind with crème fraîche, or a perfect tarte from a patisserie.

And I agree, as always, with Elizabeth David when she writes (in *Summer Cooking*) that she likes to end with a "slab of the driest, bitterest chocolate available." Green & Black's Organic is perfect.

And, finally, don't forget the corkscrew—or a bag to put the trash in.

More Useful Web Sites

www.1001huiles.fr for great vinegar and olive oil. To whet the appetite before dinner, serve chunks of Parmigiano Reggiano on a plate and gently drip their balsamic vinegar on to each piece.

www.french-truffle.com for black truffles.

www.hebrideansmokehouse.com for peat-smoked sea trout and salmon (very smoky and an acquired taste but I love it).

www.organicconsumers.org helps you find organic foods (and anything else organic come to that).

SEVEN

perfect

presents

The Pleasure of Giving

If it were not for the presents,
an elopement would be preferable.
—George Ade (1866–1944),
Forty Modern Fables

Few of us need presents but life without them would, I think, be a rather greyer matter. The instinct to give, to express one's esteem, love, affection, seems to lie deep in the human psyche. In the earliest societies the gods had to be placated with offerings. Later it was the turn of chiefs. In the poorest countries of the world people present each other with songs or flowers, little homemade bits and pieces, to indicate that they love them, think of them, admire them.

Most of us love giving presents and I can't think how we've come to the sort of state we're in in the Western world where come Christmas time they seem to be a source of such angst and resentment. If you told somebody in a poverty-stricken village in India or Africa that there were people with money and resources who yet found the buying and the choosing of presents so stressful that it kept them awake at night, and that newspapers ran dozens of articles on the subject every year, I do believe they'd conclude that we'd taken leave of our senses. And maybe we have.

Perhaps it's time to remind ourselves how lucky we are that we have money and a plethora of fabulous shops and delicious things to choose from—and, even more importantly, that we have people in our lives that we love and care about to give them to. We're short of time, I grant you, and that's a problem, but there are ways around it. One way is to pick up delightful things when we come upon them all through the year so as not to have do it all in the run-up to Christmas. For instance, I always look out for special things when I'm traveling. Every time I'm in Africa I come back with African artifacts, gorgeous wooden salad spoons or bowls, so that I've got something to give that isn't standard department store fare. In India I come back with textiles, boxes of bangles, Indian silverware, and anything else that catches my eye and that I know can't be found back home. That way I've always got something interesting and unusual ready for the occasion when a present needs to be found.

Anyway, I love presents—I love giving them, and I love getting them, though I'm usually too pressed for time to be as imaginative as I'd like to be. But it is easily observed that good presents don't need to be expensive. Recently a friend wrote and delivered a most delightful love poem for his wife's fiftieth birthday. I dare say there were a couple of more solid manifestations of his love for her as well (history does not relate), but it was the poem, read out to the assembled friends, that made her night. Another husband secretly learned to conduct a piece of music that was meaningful to him and his wife, and then conducted a small group of musicians at a party to celebrate her birthday.

One of the happiest Christmases we ever had was when our children were both at university. We rented a shooting lodge in Scotland, invited an assortment of their and our friends, and decreed that nobody was allowed to spend more than $25 on a present. It tested our ingenuity but, my goodness, we had fun—and the presents were terrific, too. I seem to remember some delicious fine olive oil, second-hand books featured largely, as did enchanting little objects found in antique shops, as well as a fantastic collection of small stationery gadgets for my home office.

The most perfect presents, of course, are those that are so particularly appropriate to the person, their life and needs, that they offer little general guidance for the rest of us. For example, the book that is perfectly chosen because it relates to something personal (the Christmas after we'd all been to Pompeii our daughter gave us Pliny the Younger's memoirs with its vivid first-person description of Vesuvius erupting—perfect) isn't quite so apt for anybody else.

I think back to the presents that have given me most pleasure: the huge Chinese pots that my husband noted I'd admired when we'd passed a shop and later bought as a surprise; the bracelets (one of chunky semiprecious stones, the other of twisted lime-green resin) that he just knew were 'me'; the little piece of embroidery my daughter did for me even though she was in the middle of intensely important exams; the Edmund de Waal series of pots that my son and daughter recently gave me as a joint birthday surprise; the special pictures my father sometimes used to give me. They're all so particular to me that it's hard to recommend them with any certainty of their being right for anybody else. So, too, the brilliant vase, bought because it will lend color and splendor to a particular room that one knows well, wouldn't go down quite so well in a totally different room with a very different aesthetic.

People with hobbies—the photographer, the football fanatic, the hiker, the tennis player, the stamp collector, the cook, the golfer—seem at first sight the easiest of all to buy things for, but the more one looks into it, the more one realizes that the more intense the relationship with the hobby, the more precision matters. The avid photographer will know precisely which lens his set is missing and something just a little bit like it won't do at all.

But as I've been giving and receiving presents for more years than I'm going to own up to, I've both given and received my share of duds. I've also had presents of such generosity and perfection that it makes me feel happy all over just thinking about them. So here are some ideas garnered from my experience of giving and receiving over the years.

For the New Mother

A night away at a ravishingly beautiful hotel (in the U.K. you might think of Olga Polizzi's ravishingly situated Endsleigh House Hotel [www.hotelendsleigh.com] in the middle of 180 acres of Devon countryside where they can sleep until noon). In the U.S. nothing could be more reviving than a couple of days at the Calistoga Ranch in the Napa Valley (580 Lommel Road, Calistoga, California 94515; www.calistogaranch.com), where there are acres of woodland, outdoor spa pools and lots of soothing Merlot. Or any other country house, hotel, or spa that's relatively easy to get to that you think would soothe and pamper.

Tickets to the opera or the theatre, paired with a night at somewhere divinely glamorous like the Waldorf (if they're traditionalists) or Gramercy Park Hotel (if they like to think they're still just a little hip), would so restore their spirits. Plus the baby-sitter.

One of Anya Hindmarch's Be a Bag bags with a picture of her baby on it. The bags are great and having a picture of the new baby makes it special (212-750-3974; www.anyahindmarch.com).

Brora's cashmere for babies (www.brora.co.uk), something from The White Company (www.thewhitecompany.co.uk), or something delicious from Baby CZ (www.babycz.com), which has lots of divine things for babies, from cashmere blankets to cute little toweling robes.

The Gigi by Storksak—the best baby hold-all in the world, according to many a new mother. Rumor has it that both Angelina Jolie and Gwyneth Paltrow have been spotted carrying one. It's really a handbag with shoulder straps and two outer pockets for all the things that Mommy needs, and a big inner pocket for all the baby stuff, with a nappy-changing pad and pockets for bottles, creams and all the rest. About $200 from www.tutti bella.com, a great Web site with lots of other ideas for mums and babies.

KidCo Peapod Portable Travel Bed folds down into a small round parcel, weighing less than ten pounds, but pops up to form a cot or safe playpen for any baby that isn't yet walking. About $50.

The Milasong hold-all-cum-suitcase called La Malice—it's brilliant for the traveling mother. It comes in three parts on a hanger, and it zips together. One section holds toys, one food, one clothes, and you simply unzip the whole thing and hang it on its hanger. You don't have to unpack or (therefore) repack—you just zip it back up again when the time comes to leave. Only, so far as I can discover, available from a few sources in France and Switzerland as well as from Pure Baby, 208 Fulham Road, London SW10 9PJ, conveniently right opposite the Chelsea & Westminster Hospital (+44 020 7751 5544; www.milasong.com). And well worth the hassle of trying to get hold of it. Delicious oils and lotions—there are so many it's hard to choose but give a generous selection of the sort of pampering bath-time pleasures that a new mother wouldn't usually buy for herself.

A half day at a spa or an appointment for a masseur, manicurist, etc., to come to the house.

A good night's sleep—if you're a godmother or grandmother, a month's maternity nurse is a fantastic present to give. Otherwise a single good night's sleep, courtesy of Gentle Hands (866-259-7659; www.gentlehandschildcare.com) gives some relief.

Give help in units of time—one hour, two hours—from a concierge service.

If you can handle shopping from QVC, the shopping channel, it has some fun things to buy. It is particularly good on girly things like great gobstopper rings for around $40 (clearly fake, or what it calls a simulated imperial topaz and pavé ring with sterling silver—but who cares?), a gorgeous "gold" bracelet consisting of lots of discs for $87, and pretty turquoise and gold-plated earrings for around $50.

For the Christening

I think there's something inherently different about a christening present. It shouldn't be ephemeral; rather it should be bought with the notion that it will be meaningful all through the child's life. And it's nicest of all if there is some real connection between the person and the presents. For instance, one of my daughter's children's godfathers—a keen fisherman—gave one of her sons a fishing rod, with the unspoken promise that he'll take him fishing later, and through the years no doubt flies and other fishing paraphernalia will also follow. It's why, of course, traditional gifts like a prayer book, Shakespeare, Dickens, and their like often appear—they're part of the background to every cultured home.

Girls are easy: little strings of tiny pearls or coral. An antique piece of jewelry or an enchanting small precious box for her to keep things in later on. Something from Tiffany, which does a great line in little silver items that aren't very expensive and come with their own beautiful boxes—silver charms, spoons, mugs, eggcups.

If you're a godparent and years of present-giving loom ahead, I think it's lovely to start a collection of something. You could do a very traditional thing and start laying down wine. Wine Cellar Services offer a great consulting service on this front (www.winecellarservices.net). It does, of course, mean that the young years should be enlivened with something else (inexpensive) come Christmas and birthdays—it's too much to expect a six-year-old to be thrilled at the prospect of waiting until he is twenty-one to enjoy his present. But when he does become twenty-one, what a thrill!

In the past I've given collections of books—the great classics, beautifully bound to make them special, and you can add to them as the years go by. The complete set of the Everyman's Library would be a great present. Its core three hundred titles represent the heart of Western literature, a platoon of living and dead writers that no other publisher can match. Rushdie, Nabokov, Dickens . . .

Something that might give a great deal of pleasure in years to come: wonderful binoculars, with the implicit promise of doing something special in later years, like going on safari.

I've also given some lovely beaten silver mugs from Nepal, one at the christening and then one each Christmas, accompanied by something cheap and cheerful on the day. You could start a collection of almost anything—precious glasses, silver, lithographs: the scope is endless.

FOR ANNIVERSARIES AND BIG "O" BIRTHDAYS

Anniversaries and big "O" birthdays are often the time when husbands and wives, fathers, mothers, and siblings give each other classic presents: a really good watch, a special camera, a fine string of pearls, a fantastic ring or brooch, some gorgeous cufflinks, the sort of things that get handed down through the generations.

But here are a few other suggestions:

The complete set of books published by Persephone. This is an enchanting small house that publishes neglected fiction, diaries, cookbooks, and short stories, all by women writers and written mainly for women, but they are all fabulous. They don't aim to be too highbrow but neither are they overtly commercial. What they do aim to do is to give real pleasure and so would provide hours and hours of delight. The Web site is www.persephonebooks.co.uk, but visit the charming little bookshop in Bloomsbury if you can, at 59 Lamb's Conduit Street, London WC1N 3NB; +44 20 7242 9292.

Photowow.com (800-453-9333) will take personal photographs and turn them into art in some way. Vacation or family photographs can be framed, set in Plexiglas, "painted" on to canvas or turned into a brilliant découpage. All the grandchildren could be photographed and turned into some art form.

Otherwise it's a good opportunity to buy something one-off and totally special, or even to commission a customized picture, piece of jewelry or silver. A fantastic black and white photograph (of the beloved, or of children, grandchildren—even a dog or horse) is a less expensive option than a portrait. You can commission an interesting piece of jewelry from most jewelers. For a portrait, contact A Stroke of Genius (727-738-1688; www.portraitartist.com), and choose the artist you like.

There are specialist galleries and craft shops all across the country that are well worth looking at because they sell things you won't find in the average chain shop or department store. A few of my favorites in London are Flow, 1–5 Needham Road, London W11 2RP, which has avant-garde tastes and beautiful things, and Contemporary Applied Art at 2 Percy Street, London W1T 1DD (www.caa.org.uk), which always has masses of one-off things—almost all hotly desirable, in glass, ceramics, jewelry, textiles.

Maureen Doherty of Egg has a brilliant eye and her small craft gallery at 36–37 Kinnerton Street, London SW1X 8ES, often has beautiful, special things, including silver work by William Welstead, and she also has some lovely unpolished diamond necklaces (not expensive).

Commission a special binding for a favorite book. Get a first edition, if you can, and then consult www.bookarts.com for a bookbinder to customize it. The Web site has details of individual bookbinders as well as sensible advice.

THE THANK-YOU PRESENT

I've been musing on the matter of what constitutes the perfect weekend house (or country villa or yacht) present. Unless we're like Uncle Matthew in Nancy Mitford's *Love in a Cold Climate,* who never liked to go anywhere (least of all, of course, abroad), we none of us want—do we?—to be like the man who was invited to most of the grand houses of the country—just once. Though whether it was due to something he said or the presents he took isn't clear. If we are lucky to be invited to share our friends' country cottages, tennis courts, swimming pools, and herbaceous borders, clearly we cannot arrive empty-handed.

Take your hostess or host luxurious versions of everyday things—a new or particularly lovely version of bath oils and gorgeous soaps.

Softly padded exquisite hangers—Laura Ashley does lovely ones. A beautiful pair of pillowcases, antique if possible and only in white.

A single perfect silver jam spoon, butter knife, horn spoon for caviar, honey spoon or big serving spoon or salad servers, from a specialist craft shop or maker, or from an antique shop.

Other things that have gone down well: the latest hardback biography or must-read novel; a luscious gardening tome (if they're into gardening); a beautiful (antique or wonderfully carved modern) doorstop.

Food treats: a round of cheddar, a big chunk of real parmesan, a jar of saffron, *bottarga* (that fabulous dried tuna's roe that is ambrosia folded into pasta), a bottle of truffle oil, olive oils and balsamic vinegars with a special provenance. A great knife, a beautifully packaged game. Chocolates, but only if they're really good; a box of Russell Stover's won't do. Truffles from one of the small artisanal chocolate houses popping up everywhere would be fantastic. A magnum of fine wine (much nicer, says my friend with the smart Scottish shooting lodge, than supermarket champagne). Addresses of good foodie Web sites are all to be found in chapter 6 (see page 303).

Gardening presents—if they have gardens—obviously need to suit the garden and the gardeners, but Outsidepride .com has a tub of mixed seeds for wild flowers to attract butterflies, bees, and birds. At $15.99 for enough to cover a hundred square feet.

The most imaginative present I ever heard of was that of an expert gardener who took to a less horticulturally gifted friend fifty rare and precious tulip bulbs and planted them all herself. Antonia Fraser was once on the receiving end (though no doubt not from a house guest) of a rose hedge: "a daily renewed present," as she put it.

Authentic gardening tubs, a linen tool bag, oilskin or leather kneeling pads, exceptionally sturdy glass storm lanterns, twine dispenser, mini bocci boules or a croquet set all make good presents, and can be found at R. K. Alliston (www.rkalliston.com).

A friend who owns a house in France said that one of the nicest presents she was ever given was a beautifully bound album filled with photographs of the holiday that they'd all shared, which arrived a week or two after the visit. Another friend, a very successful property developer, took a whole group of friends to St. Petersburg for his fiftieth and one of the party put together a wonderful album, full of photographs, drawings, stickers and anecdotes, to commemorate the event. Those are presents that are infinitely precious because they show thought, take time and care, and are so particular and personal. *And,* take note, do not cost a fortune.

The Wedding Present

Trickier and trickier. . . . These days so many couples are getting married so much later by which time they've got not just one, but two sets of all the things once found on traditional wedding lists. That doesn't mean to say that there isn't scope for beautiful, upgraded versions of some of the useful household accoutrements—really ravishing serving spoons, silver, glass, linen, candlesticks, and all the rest. But taste and lifestyle have such an important part to play that it's hard to give one-size-fits-all advice. If we're lucky, the bride and groom will guide us. When Lady Sarah Chatto, Princess Margaret's daughter, got married, I seem to remember she asked for nothing but books. That would send one scurrying off to find special editions or perhaps sourcing a complete set of a beautiful edition of something like Dickens or an author you know the couple particularly love.

I think that on the whole, unless you are very close to the couple and really understand their taste, it's best to give what I call taste-neutral presents, or to consult the wedding list if there is one, which will at least give you some idea of where their tastes lie. The quirky candlesticks that you absolutely love may clash, not just with their own inclinations but with the candlesticks and the house they already have. If they're really close—like your children, a godchild or a best friend—then something special, chosen with care from an antique shop, a small interior design shop like some of those listed in chapter 5, or a special craft shop, makes a terrific present, as they won't have anything else like it. For those less close to the happy couple, my advice is to keep it more neutral.

More Ideas

A fantastic case of fine wine. Either your local wine merchant or somebody like Wine Cellar Services (www.winecellar services.net) will give good advice, and will also help you find a place to store the wine if the couple haven't got anywhere to keep it until it's ready to drink.

The best food mixer—say, the original Waring mixer (if they haven't got one and if you know they're cooks).

His and hers plain white bathrobes. Gorgeous thick white towels, or some great beach towels.

A fantastic set of kitchen knives plus a sharpener, from Williams-Sonoma (www.williams-sonoma.com).

A really fine leather photograph album or visitors' book, from Smythson (www.smythson.com).

A set of amazing saucepans, from Alessi, 130 Greene Street, New York, NY 10012.

Carl Rotter water glasses in jewel colors from www.arte dona.com.

Some antique glasses—a pair, or a set of six or eight, for water, wine, or champagne.

A great espresso machine—a Gaggia (nice and plain and classic) for choice.

For Him

Bamford & Sons, whose flagship store is in London at 31 Sloane Square, (+44 20 7881 8010) has now arrived at Bergdorf Goodman's in New York (and at www.bamfordandsons.com) and it has to be one of the most irresistible shops in the world for men. It doesn't go in for gimmicks and flashy eye-catching touches but instead homes in on all those absolutely classic things that most of the men I know love—soft-as-butter cashmere scarves, light-as-a-feather cashmere jackets, relaxed leather jackets, deep grey flannel trousers, gorgeous leather gloves and satchels—but gives them all a relaxed and modern twist.

Fabulous toys for the boys make great presents. . . . Track down divine tiny (three-inch) digital cameras, which have all the newfangled technology (SD memory cards, white balance, fast shutter speeds, two-megapixel sensors and LCD monitors) but look exactly like a miniature old-fashioned Rolleiflex Twin Reflex camera. Or the brilliant OQO Mini Computer Notebook, which, since it isn't cheap, is probably mainly of interest to the city bonus crowd. It's easily portable (it weighs less than a pound) and has "Wifi, Bluetooth, 30gb shock-mounted HDD, and an easy docking solution." It means you can send and read e-mails, you can listen to music on a train or watch a movie on a plane. It also has a proper keyboard concealed under a slide-out screen.

A vintage Rolex can be bought from the Vintage Watch Company, 24 Burlington Arcade, London W1J 0EA (+44 20 7499 2032 and at www.vintagewatchcompany.com) or in the United States from Robert Maron (www.robertmaron.com).

Moleskin notebooks, the ones allegedly used by Bruce Chatwin and Ernest Hemingway, from Modo e Modo, make a terrific small present. Get the authentic article from virtually any bookstore or your local stationer.

Personalize the selection for his iPod if he hasn't got around to doing it himself . . . with sentimental songs for an anniversary.

A DVD of the Super Bowl.

A masseur to come to the house and give ten massages (this was my last birthday present to my husband, and he loved it).

Transparent shower-proof speakers so he can sing along as he soaps.

Clothes

These are always tricky, but I haven't known too many men who don't love a bespoke shirt from Seize Sur Vingt in New York (243 Elizabeth Street, New York 10012; 212-343-0476) or from Emmett (380 King's Road, London SW3 5U2; +44 20 7351 7529; www.emmettlondon.com), cashmere socks (for winter treats) and soft-as-butter napa gloves from Ralph Lauren or Bill Amberg (230 Elizabeth Street, New York 10012; 212-625-9565; www.billamberg.com), ties by Paul Smith (108 Fifth Avenue, New York 10011; 212-627-9770), fine-gauge silky knits by John Smedley (at Barney's) and cashmere sweaters from Asprey (853 Madison Avenue, New York 10021; 212-688-1811; www.asprey.com). Not to mention an original Belstaff jacket.

FOR KIDS

Some of the best presents for children that I've found take imagination. For instance, for one grandson's birthday we bought him a backpack and filled it with survival aids: a two-way walkie-talkie, a small flashlight, a small multipurpose knife, a water bottle, a book on edible plants and flowers, and so on, all bought from a selection of camping shops, like REI or Cabela's. He keeps it in his family's farmhouse in France and takes it with him when they go for all-day walks. My mother gave my daughter when she was small a tiny, colorful chest of drawers, each drawer tissue-lined and with some treat inside it—a small bracelet, some colored pencils, and so on.

The Museum of Natural History is a great source of presents with lots of books, puzzles and kits based on dinosaurs, skeletons to put together, scientific experiments to do. In fact most museums are great for interesting presents and if you aren't near a museum most malls have a branch of the Nature Store which has some terrific scientific, eco-presents for kids.

There are lovely small children's shops tucked away all over the country, which those of you who live near them know all about. But for those who don't fancy the nightmare that a visit to FAO Schwarz entails, wonderful though their departments are (the traffic, the lack of parking, the crowds: the full disaster), it's worth knowing that there are lots of great Web sites where all you have to do is browse, sit back, and your chosen item will be sent to you.

Web Sites for Kids' Presents

American Girl (www.americangirl.com) is a mecca for little girls. Lots of beautiful dolls with coordinating clothing, books, movies, and accessories. American Girl Place, found in many cities such as Atlanta, Dallas, Chicago, Los Angeles, and New York. New York has shopping, dining, live musicals, all designed to appeal to little girls. The American Girl Boutique and Bistro has a special selection of the dolls, books, and outfits with casual dining and American Girl–themed celebrations for birthday parties.

Kitson kids, online (www.shopkitson.com) and on Robertson Boulevard in Los Angeles, is very celebrity, chic, cool, funky. Children's clothing, accessories, toys. Popular with the stars . . . very kitsch.

www.boomerangtoys.com is "Just what a toy store should be," according to the "Zagat Survey 2007: Best Stores in New York City" (New York City)—that says it all.

www.mcphee.com has inexpensive, silly joke toys, stickers, and candies. They even have a Carl Jung action figure!

www.metmuseum.org/store. This is a great source of children's toys—lots are very beautiful, with fantastic pop-up books and art and science related presents. It's ranked highly by Zagat and Forbes. There are twenty-three Met stores in premier malls, airports, and exclusive locations across the United States in Arizona, California, Colorado, Florida, Georgia, Massachusetts, Nevada, New Jersey, New York, and Texas. The Metropolitan also has seventeen stores around the world in Australia, Austria, India, Japan, Mexico, Singapore, and Thailand.

www.fao.com is a really terrific toy store with the sort of things that can't be found in your average chain store. Filled with every manner of toy from the smallest to those "hard-to-find and oh-so-expensive items like Vespa scooters for older children, mini luxury cars like Hummers and Jaguars, and serious karaoke machines," as *Frommer's Review* puts it. There's also a soda fountain where the kids can load up on sugar and the giant piano keys made famous in the movie *Big* are still in place. A brilliant Web site. It will shortly embark on a project to put its toy stores in 685 Macy's department stores.

www.dylanscandybar.com. All kids—not to mention their parents—love these stores, which were founded by Ralph Lauren's daughter, Dylan. They're wonderfully bright and upbeat and besides almost every conceivable kind of candy sell a small range of clothes, jewelry, and toys.

For a Young Boy

Movie gift certificate card from AMC Theatres (www.amc theatres.com).

Football table from $600.

Foldaway hammock.

A globe light.

CBGB T-shirts from www.cbgb.com.

Pepe jeans.

Games: air hockey table, or a Batman pinball or a Laser FX Bowling Arcade Game or a darts set, with board and cabinet.

Travel speakers for his iPod and a pack of six iPod socks.

FOR
MISCELLANEOUS BIRTHDAYS
AND ANNIVERSARIES

A sundial or sculpture for the garden.

Gourmet food basket.

A first edition of a favorite novel, such as *Oranges Are Not the Only Fruit* by Jeanette Winterson, from a used bookstore. Price depends upon condition.

Now that smoothies are what the health-conscious set are drinking, a KitchenAid Ultra Power blender from Macy's.

Track down wonderful old planters or vintage receptacles and fill them with bulbs ready to bloom in the spring.

Recorded Books, great for long car journeys or for those whose eyes are no longer what they were, from www.recorded books.com.

Customized stationery, from www.crane.com.

A few fashion-y ideas for a young girl: a leather Filofax, a funky watch (by Dolce & Gabbana), beatnik tights, a manicure kit, and Chanel lip gloss.

Tickets for ice skating at Rockefeller Center.

Silk pajamas from Carine Gilson, at Agent Provocateur (7961 Melrose Avenue, Los Angeles 90046; 323-653-0229) and at www.carinegilson.com.

Antiques, being one-offs, always make terrific presents. Antique spoons, bowls, jars—for instance one perfect antique Blanc de China rice bowl or a large temple jar.

Cute customized cashmere sweaters. Jeanetta Rowan-Hamilton takes old cashmere sweaters (much better quality than new ones, she says) and gives them new life by adding lace, buttons, frills, embroidery—they're quirky and delicious (+44 20 7584 3030 and at www.nettlescashmere.com).

For Those
Awkward People
Who Have Everything

Giving presents used to be a breeze. A new handbag, cashmere socks, a brilliant little gadget, a fine new saucepan, some fabulous scent, if carefully matched to the nearest and dearest, could usually be guaranteed to bring a smile to the face and a thank-you letter in the mail. These days, though, giving presents is infinitely more taxing. Most of us, even those of us who are far from rich, have way too much stuff. We can identify with David Collins, the interior designer, when he said, "I really can't wear another pair of shoes or carry another bag."

What all this boils down to is that we need to think harder, plan more and add a huge dollop of imagination into the mix. Not easy. So here are a few suggestions as to what might go down well for those who really have no need of another pair of socks, a coffret of lotions and potions, or even a "must-have" handbag or designer suit. Some of them are expensive (aimed at that annoying fellow who "has everything"), but not all—and if you're prepared to do the work yourself (sort the iPod, make the memory box, cook the special meal), then they can be relatively cheap.

And if you're really stuck you could do what my husband did for a recent big birthday of my own (I think he'd surveyed the house and the wardrobe and given up on the whole notion of any more "things"). He arranged instead for the scattered immediate family to be together for the whole day and organized a series of not very expensive treats (a trip up the London Eye, lunch in a Chinese restaurant, a visit to a cinema followed by a special tea). It couldn't have been nicer.

1. Sort the iPod. For the technophobe who wants to load his iPod and doesn't know how, www.audiosushi.net will do it for you. It will put together a specially customized playlist of music and, for $100 to $150, give an hour's personal tutoring in how to download music and manage the program. For $175 to $260 they'll devise an eighty-minute playlist, put the music on your iPod or on your mp3 player.

2. Frame the album covers. For a music lover—particularly a fan of pop music—get the best old album covers framed. Gives a wonderful chart of the musical history of the recipient.

3. Horticulture. An avenue of trees, a sea of daffodils, a hedge of roses: presents to last forever. A tree-lined avenue of ten flame-shaped hornbeams (*Carpinus betulus*) would be about $8,000 (£4,000). A five-acre sea of daffodils could be done for £8,000. A five-acre rolled "instant" summer-flowering meadow would be £27,000, while a five-meter run of pleached magnolias could be done for £2,500 and a hedge of hybrid tea rose bushes (Rosa 'Black Baccarat') for £450. Your very own award-winning Chelsea flower show garden would be £250,000. All from Woodhams Landscape (+44 20 7730 3353 and at www.woodhams.co.uk). Remember, you don't have to get the professionals in. Do the planning yourself and it's not only more meaningful, but also much less expensive.

4. A special weekend. Fly by jet to Venice for a private after-hours tour of St. Mark's Basilica. Go by gondola to a private candlelit palace, be serenaded by world-class opera singers, and have dinner prepared by a top Italian chef: from about $17,000 per person.

Three nights in Florence. Stay at the Ferragamo family private palace on the Arno. Day 1: Dine at Enoteca Pinchiorri with a set menu *degustazione* for two people at one of the best restaurants in Italy with outstanding food and a fantastic wine list. Day 2: A tailor from Ermenegildo Zegna, one of Italy's top menswear brands, will send a tailor to your penthouse suite to offer its made-to-measure service (the suit is included in the price). A private visit with a guide to the Vasari Corridor, running from the Uffizi to the Pitti Palace, over the Ponte Vecchio, with an unrivalled collection of portraits. Day 3: A convertible Alfa Romeo Giulietta is delivered to the hotel for a drive through the rolling Tuscan countryside to the Cappezine estate, home of Avignonesi, one of the finest vineyards in Italy. There's a private tour of the cellars and vineyards, then a four-course lunch and wine-tasting in the loggia overlooking the hill town of Montepulciano. Day 4: a hot-air balloon ride taking off at dawn from the olive groves of Montisi. A champagne breakfast greets you on touchdown. A Mercedes with private driver takes you to and from the airport or the station. From about $9,000 per person.

Both available from Bellini Travel (www.bellinitravel.com).

5. A pair of swans, for the must-have lake. You can buy different types from Knox Swan & Dog (www.canadiangoose control.com)—black-neck swans are relatively inexpensive, as are whooper swans, and at the more expensive end are mute swans and trumpeters. If hatchlings are available, Knox offers a same-day delivery service across the country. Call them at 847-304-1230.

Swans, though, are not very biddable so bear in mind that they have been known to abscond to other more favorable lakes.

6. The special book. For a first wedding anniversary a doting husband found a first edition of *Rebecca* by Daphne du Maurier (a favorite of his wife), arranged for Joan Fontaine (who starred in the film) to sign it and then got it specially bound. A wife found a first edition of *The Compleat Angler* (for $50,000 plus) for a fishing-mad husband. If you want to find a first-edition book, start at www.abebooks.com, a Canadian-run site that began as a book exchange and now carries stocklists for rare book collectors and sellers around the world. Bertram Rota, which stocks modern first-edition books from 1890, will conduct more complicated searches for books (+44 20 7836 0723 and at www.bertramrota.co.uk).

Maggs Bros Rare Books (www.maggs.com) has a large collection of first-edition books. Simon Finch (who recently sold a Shakespeare first folio edition for $2.4 million) is another dealer in rare books (www.simonfinch.com).

7. Commission a symphony. Follow in the footsteps of Mervyn King, governor of the Bank of England, and Sir Nicholas Goodison, ex-chairman of the Stock Exchange. King contacted the London Symphony Orchestra and, with six friends, commissioned a symphony. It cost them over $35,000 over three years ($6,000 per head), but they had creative control over the project and worked with players from the orchestra. A cheaper alternative is offered by the Birmingham Contemporary Music Group: as a Sound Investor for $200, you can buy a share in a symphony or you can buy the entire symphony for from $20,000. When it is ready, you get to attend rehearsals, go to the première, meet the composer and get a signed copy of the score (www.bcmg.org.uk).

8. Handmade model of a house. David Linley will create a model of your humble cottage, fine rectory, beautiful manor house or very grand castle. (Castle Howard, done as a present for Simon Howard, its owner, is just one of his many commissions.) From around £25,000 ($50,000). It can be entirely decorative or made into the form of a humidor, jewelry, or pencil case (+44 20 7730 7300 and at www.davidlinley.com).

9. A special day with a sports, literary, or culinary hero. Play a game of tennis with John McEnroe or a round of golf with Greg Norman. The cost of the game depends upon the star—and is rising all the time.

Have lunch at a top restaurant with a literary figure such as Martin Amis, Margaret Atwood, Zadie Smith, or Roddy Doyle, from £5,000 ($10,000).

A famous chef to cook at home: Raymond Blanc, Anthony Worrall-Thompson, Ainsley Harriott, Rick Stein, and many others. The price depends on who the chef is. From around £15,000 ($30,000).

Quintessentially will organize any of the above once you join (www.quintessentially.com).

10. A day with a personal shopper. Choose from Paris, New York, London, Delhi, or Bombay. Whisk him or her there by private jet.

In Paris, Susan Tabak's your woman. She's best of friends with some of the capital's sassiest dressers (Nathalie Rykiel,

Loulou de la Falaise, Marie-Hélène de Taillac, to name but three). From $1,500 a day (212-404-8398 and at www.paris personalshopper.com).

In London Nicola Robinson, who works for a specialist company called Being Seen, offers her limousine-driven services at $150 an hour—contact her at info@beingseen.co.uk.

In Bombay, Greaves Travel (888-414-0333) can fix for Monica Vaziralli to find you the finest pashminas, best-value diamonds, sumptuous silks and off-beat antiques. A three-day package, flying out on Thursday night, arriving back at seven A.M. on Monday with two days with a private shopper and a luxury car.

In New York, stay at the Mandarin Oriental and book four hours with a personal shopper at Bergdorf Goodman or organize Kathleen Beckett, formerly with *Vogue* magazine (212-505-2157 or info@BeckettsBlackBook.com), who for a straight charge of $250 an hour will take you shopping, not just to ordinary shops but to the designers themselves, to small little-known boutiques, to "the king of trousers," to the best costume jeweler, to cult names where she negotiates sizeable discounts. "I've never had a client yet who hasn't saved my fee by lunch-time."

Plants and Flowers

A bunch of flowers every week of the year must be one of the best presents ever—expensive but memorable. Scented roses can be delivered every month from Calyx Flowers (800-800-7788 and at www.calyxflowers.com) at $549.95 for a year's worth. www.jane-carroll.com is a wonderful Web site delivering fresh flowers, brilliantly arranged, all over the United States.

New York isn't short of fantastic florists and sometimes a bunch of simple roses or tulips looks better than anything more elaborate. Takashimaya Floral Boutique (693 Madison Avenue, 212-350-0111) has one of the most seductive flower shops in the world, while Wild Poppy (159 East Ninety-second Street 212-717-5757), Elizabeth Ryan (411 East Ninth Street, 212-995-1111); and Spruce (222 Eighth Avenue, 212-929-9252) all can be trusted to send the sort of flowers you'd like to be receiving yourself.

Special Florists Around the World

Paris: Christian Tortu is the most famous Parisian florist, at 6 Carrefour de l'Odéon, 75006 Paris (+33 1 43 26 02 56).

London: Wild at Heart (+44 20 7727 3095); Ercole Moroni at McQueen's (+44 20 7251 5505); Orlando Hamilton (+44 20 8962 8944); Rob van Helden (+44 20 7720 6774 and at www.partyflowers-london.co.uk).

CHARITABLE PRESENTS

Amongst the very well-heeled set and the not-so-young crowd, it is now quite the norm to ask either for no presents or to suggest a charity for guests to donate to instead. Many people have their own favorite charities and sometimes a specific one is named. Otherwise, choose one that means something special to the couple getting married.

Or give to eco-charities like Earthroots (www.earthroots .org) and get a great gift for your budding animal lover.

Adopt a Wolf for just $25 (www.wolfhaven.org).

Through the World Wildlife Fund (www.worldwildlife .org), you can organize to adopt any number of endangered species—a tiger, gorilla, polar bear, panda.

It's also very fashionable these days to ask wedding guests to contribute to environmental charities, most particularly when they've been asked to fly hundreds of miles to the wedding itself. www.carbonneutral.com (which used to be called Future Forests) enables you to buy trees to reforest a big selection of projects.

Through www.rainforestforever.com you can adopt a tree in the Brazilian rainforest, for which you get a certificate plus a map showing the exact location where your tree is planted.

Through Oxfam Unwrapped (www.oxfamamericaunwrapped .com) plant fifty trees.

Robin Birley (whose father Mark Birley famously founded Annabel's, Harry's Bar, and Mark's Club) started www.enviro trade.co.uk, which develops projects in Mozambique that encourage the local population to treasure their forests. You can buy carbon credits via the Web site.

WRAPPING

I'm of the school of thought that thinks that wrapping matters. I'm entranced by lovely packaging and one of the great joys of visiting Japan is the sheer aesthetic refinement of it all. A single apple is wrapped and then delivered to its buyer with all the care and love that in the United States might be attached to buying jewels. Do I always manage, come Christmastime, to deliver up little works of wrapped art? Of course not. But, unless something is oversized (which, funnily enough, many children's presents tend to be, the bicycle, the doll's house, the foosball table) they at least get wrapped somehow. And I do have aspirations—one day, one Christmas, it's all going to be gorgeous. In the meantime, for those who are really pushed for time, more and more stores offer wrapping services, which, when you're lucky enough to have lots of people you care about to find presents for, is, one has to confess, an amazing boon.

For a particular birthday, you can go to town because there are just one or two presents to consider. Color combinations, paper, ribbons, and trimmings can all be customized and time taken. You could choose papers that are somehow specific—special newspapers or maps; or ordinary white paper with photographs printed digitally on them; a music score of a piece of music that is meaningful. Try customizing the container, for instance, matching it to something imaginative: flower pots for something horticultural, cake tins for something food-related—you get the idea. You can make the package seem special by adding little stars, flowers, beads.

Come Christmas, I usually adopt a streamlined approach. I have a color scheme each year and everybody's present gets the same wrapping. Funnily enough, it works quite well because, when all the family is together and everything is piled up under the tree, it makes the groups easily identifiable. One ploy could be to use a different color scheme for each family group, making it easier to distribute them.

I've used plain brown paper in the past, which can look wonderfully chic particularly if you use a nice wide black ribbon. I quite often use plain silver paper with gold ribbon or plain gold with silver ribbon. Both gold and silver, if plain, also look gorgeous with any jewel-colored ribbon and make a happy background for stars and other stickers.

In India I sometimes fall in love with their gorgeous hand-made papers but they don't work very well for wrapping—they're too stiff and not malleable enough. But tissue paper works well and if, on Christmas Eve, you run out of paper, you can always use tinfoil, though it is a little on the fragile side.

Newspaper is another useful emergency wrapping and it can be saved from looking tatty by folding the edges and using some wide black ribbon—very graphic.

Don't stint on buying paper, it's foolish. If you buy too much, you can use it up during the year or at the following Christmas, but if you don't have enough on Christmas Eve you're stuck. Keep ribbons as they come in during the year and recycle them. These days you can buy cute boxes and bags that make good containers for presents. Kate's Paperie, 561 Broadway, New York, (and check www.katespaperie.com for its other branches) has fabulous paper and special ribbons, too.

Stock up on supplies if you ever go to India, most particularly in Delhi, where you should go to Chandni Chowk, where they sell a myriad wonderful things for every kind of festivity for literally a few pennies. I buy ribbons and all sorts of glittery bits and pieces—flowers, stars, beads, plastic drops, decorations—to bring home and put in the Christmas drawer.

Favorite Places to Buy Wrapping Around the World

U.K.

Paperchase, 213–215 Tottenham Court Road, London WC2 7PS (www.paperchase.co.uk), has a fantastic selection of papers, labels, tags, boxes and bags.

Temptation Alley, 359–361 Portobello Road, London W10 5SA (www.temptationalley.com), is a gem, filled with all sorts of decorative ideas from feathers, buttons, fabrics—you name it.

V. V. Rouleaux must be one of my favorite shops of all time. It is filled with decorative inspiration—ribbons, bows, butterflies, flowers. Check it all out on www.vvrouleaux.com.

The Wrapping Company, (+44 1483 823 023 and at www .thewrappingco.com), has lots of cute bags for bottles, chic boxes for everything from a cashmere sweater to a pair of cuff links, masses of tags and a vast variety of ribbons.

ITALY

Italy has fabulous papers of all kinds, including beautiful hand-marbled ones—a little expensive if you're doing lots of wrapping but lovely for a one-off treat.

Il Papiro, check www.ilpapirofirenze.it for branches. They are all over Italy with six branches in Florence and four in Venice.

TOKYO

Tokyo Kyukyodo, 5-7-4, Ginza Chuo-ku, has a fantastic selection of Japanese paper products. Whether it's a little notebook, some writing paper, a cute bookmark, an address book or fanciful paper creations, they're all beautiful.

A FEW GOOD WEB SITES
FOR PRESENTS

www.raptdirect.com (+44 870 160 7580). An offshoot of OKA, a charming provider of decorative pieces for the home, Rapt is a small mail-order or online operation that is geared specifically to the market for presents. Nothing dramatic, but the sort of pieces that would fit into most people's homes: big hurricane lights, small leather-covered tape measures, throws (nicely Eastern, with a touch of Paisley), Nailsea wine glasses, candlesticks—you get the picture.

www.redenvelope.com is a really good source of presents that most of us would like—terrific candles, candle-holders, photograph frames . . . that sort of thing.

www.reglisse.co.uk is run by Pascale Karam-Boemond, a chic Lebanese who lived in Paris for years, and she has things you won't find in most shops—Gaetano Pesce's amazing resin vases-cum-sculptures, jewelry by Philippe Ferrandis, who makes jewelry for many of the haute couture houses, ceramics from a Danish design duo, one of whom helped modernize the grand old house of Copenhagen China. She's got a great eye and great taste.

www.notonthehighstreet.com brings together a whole range of niche designers and craftspeople. Search for quirky bags and jewelry, for offbeat craft items and, one thing's for sure, you won't find them in any of the major department stores.

www.plumo.com is another enchanting little catalogue and online source of things you won't see anywhere else. It has a rather rustic, nostalgic air to it and is definitely not for city slickers, but if you're looking for a flower-spattered silk ki-mono, some embroidered handkerchiefs (oooh, that takes me back), some adorable little pagoda lanterns or some pressed glass cake stands, then Plumo will come up trumps.

EIGHT

❦

fun

and

games

PARTIES

Elsa Maxwell was a legendary party giver in the 1930s, featuring regularly in magazines such as *Vogue* and all the newspapers society pages, but if one listened to her advice, nobody would ever dare give one. I can't believe it's *that* tricky myself. But I do go along with her when she says that no hostess (to use the vocabulary of her heyday) should take her own party so seriously that the guests end up being solemn about it as well. The best parties are gifts to your friends. The point of a party is to have fun.

Most of us have been to the sort of party that is more of an ordeal than a pleasure—the sort where nobody introduces you to anybody and you mill about, having to make your way through a mêlée of heaving bodies, hoping desperately to catch the eye of somebody you know. It seems to be a formula that some people indulge in at New Year's Eve, where your hosts keep you standing around with nothing more substantial than endless drinks until midnight, when they finally produce something long after one is past it, and never introduce you to anybody.

Speaking personally, I've always loved best the sort of party where you eventually sit down—where there are perhaps drinks first and then a proper placement so you really do get to meet at least your neighbors properly. I love small dinner parties and anything where there is a possibility of genuine exchange. I also love the sort of parties that people are more prone to give around Christmastime when all the generations are mixed up and our hosts include both their children and their parents. Games are played with everybody mixing in and such parties often end the evening with carols around the piano. And then, of course, there is the grand party to mark an engagement, a wedding, an anniversary—the tent, the setting, the band and the dancing. They can be wonderful, provided the hosts have done more than worry about the theme, the food and the decor, and have gone to the trouble of thinking who might like to sit next to whom, organizing the table plans with real care.

I'm not particularly adventuresome myself since our house, being long and thin without one single room large enough for more than about twenty-five people, doesn't lend itself to parties but I've been to enough to know what works from the guests' point of view. I'm with Elsa Maxwell when she says: "A good party should occur in one room only, and that room should always be too small." (But only just too small; very much too small, which I've also experienced, doesn't work either because you can't circulate and you get trapped.)

The best parties have an entertaining mix of guests but I have this old-fashioned notion that parties are for your friends, so the idea (much promoted by professional party givers) of inviting famous people one doesn't know to jazz up the proceedings is, to my mind, bizarre. Beauties, eccentrics, creative people, and great entertainers are all great additions to the mix—if you happen to have them in your circle. In my view, it's critical to try to think who might be pleased to meet one another, and to make sure you introduce people likely to get along. The really big sin in my book is merely to throw yourself into enjoying your own party while giving no thought as to how your guests are doing (and, believe me, I've been to a few like that).

In our early married days, rather Spartan parties were the order of the day, but since the advent of proper party planners and fancy caterers, the ante has been upped considerably. Wedding parties take place in Rome and Prague, in castles and on tropical islands, and the celebrations are meticulously planned over many days. (Did the Hurley/Nayar celebrations really take eight days?) I don't recall much in the way of bachelorette parties, baby showers or Halloween parties when I was growing up, but these days they're all the rage. Even children's parties have become a source of angst with tiny tots demanding to know what the entertainment is (in my day, you made your own and Grandmother's Whispers—or Telephone—was our idea of a great game), while goody bags, getting fatter and more luxurious by the day, on departure are, it seems, de rigueur. No wonder it's become a stressful matter.

Which is why if the party is going to be large and grand, there's nothing for it but to hand it over to the professionals. If you're strapped for cash or want to do it simply, you can buy in bits of help. You can hire simple tents—just Google "rent a tent" and you're spoiled for choice. Prices vary hugely depending upon the grandeur and elaboration of the tent itself and of the decorations inside. If you live in the country you can often get local women to do some of the food while you rope in friends and family to do, say, the flowers and the puddings.

For dinner parties at home I often have some help. We have an open-plan kitchen and dining room, so there's no room for staff, as there's no behind-the-scenes place to put them. There was a time when I knew of a wonderful girl who would cook the entire dinner party at her home and deliver it to me at six o'clock on the given day with precise instructions as to how to serve it and what needed heating, and with all the garnishes in sweet little containers. Alas, she's gone the way of such help and has got married, giving dinner parties of her own. But I still buy in odd bits of help. I quite often order the first and last courses and do the main course myself. If you're in New York you can call Zabar's (212-496-1234; www.zabars .com).

Or you can hand over the party arrangements lock, stock, and barrel. Party planners these days are increasingly inventive and they not only come up with themes but have all the props to bring the theme to life. I once saw the warehouse of John Robertson-Roxborough (of the first-class caterers the Admirable Crichton), and it was huge, so stuffed to the gills with endless varieties of glasses, flower containers, tablecloths, tables, and a host of other paraphernalia, that you could see why he is able to conjure up so many different sorts of magic. As to themes, financier Ben Goldsmith had an ice cavern for his twenty-first; Elton and David like to go in for kings and queens and their opulence themes; Truman Capote famously had a black-and-white ball; Patti and Andy Wong every Chinese New Year ask their friends to dress up according to the particular theme of the ball; one hedge-fund manager had a heaven and hell party (which sounds rather fun: guests could wander between the two).

I think seating plans matter hugely. It's an act of generosity and essential to a good party to try to match people who might like each other, fall in love with each other or just have a rattling good conversation. Some people like switching the seating plan halfway through a dinner, getting the men to move along a few paces. I rather like that, though to be sure sometimes you've just got going when it's time to move on. Husbands and wives or other couples should be on different tables at large parties but if they are at the same table do not seat them next to each other—they can do that at home and it isn't why they've come. Don't put best friends together either; they see each other all the time, too. At big seated dinners the host and hostess should make a point of visiting all the tables, checking that all is well and nobody seems left out.

Whom to put next to the host is a tricky question. You can choose the most cheerful, amusing person there, but I think it displays better manners to look after those who might know the fewest people, who are very old or who have come the farthest distance. I remember being immensely touched at a very, very grand summer lunch party being put on the right hand of our host when there were many much more important people there. It showed exquisite manners, for he realized that my husband and I were less likely than most to know many people there (they were new friends of ours and it was the first time we had been invited to their house), and he did it (I assume) to make sure we were properly looked after. These are the sort of manners that come from an inner courtesy and elegance, and are what one hopes for in a perfect host.

☞ *I think friends rather like being asked to help at a party. Some could pour drinks and make sure everybody's glass is full, and others introduce people who seem to be out on a limb or on their own.*

VENUE

Of course it depends on the party. Small ones—dinner parties, small birthday parties—are nicest at home. For anything bigger, and for people with country cottages or houses and lawns, the simplest solution is to hire a tent. You might think about combining a couple of parties—we've been to many a friend's big "O" or wedding anniversary party where either the night before or the night after, a child has its twenty-first birthday party. But there are all sorts of unordinary places for hire for parties, ranging from historic estates and gardens to clubs and theaters. Most caterers have lists of suitable venues, but some of the options are the Smithsonian Museum, the Ferry Building in San Francisco, the Central Park Zoo and the Biltmore Estates, not to mention some offbeat venues, such as the Beckham Creek Cave House (888-371-2283), which is a wonderful if bizarre venue for a wedding or other party. The list is endless, not to mention the large number of country estates and islands that can be hired in every corner of the country, plus castles both small and large abroad.

ATMOSPHERE

Lighting is important. Anything too harsh spoils the atmosphere. At a big dinner, groups of small candles—votives—are wonderful. You can group them on tables or side tables around the house. At night you can add lots of enchantment to the proceedings by lighting up the steps to the house on both sides. I've seen paper bags used as containers with tea-lights inside them. Some versions are made of fire-retardant white paper, or have a pretty etched pattern in them that is illuminated once a tea-light is put inside. Put lights in the trees if you have them or hang lanterns, or stick huge garden torches in the ground to light up a drive or pathway. To lend magic to the garden there are now little battery-operated lights that need no electricity. Gaiam (877-989-6321 and at www.gaiam.com) sells battery-operated hummingbirds, butterflies, and dragonflies that are mounted on black sticks so that they appear invisible at night. You simply stick them into flowerpots or into the earth so that they appear to hover. Should you happen to have a pond, a lake, or a still river, you could add magic with floating water lily lights that have an LED inside them so that the light changes as it glows.

Strings of pretty lights that can be draped over mirrors or the edges of tables can be found in most housewares stores these days. They need to be plugged into an electrical socket but they add a lot of magic and come in various forms (flowers, stars, blossoms). You can also drape coiled lights in Muji's transparent cubes at Christmas.

For dinner parties, lots of candles are wonderful. Massed ranks of assorted candlesticks, hurricane lamps, or candelabra all would look good.

Flowers are, of course, essential for the good party, and if you're doing a large party with caterers, you'll probably get the flowers done by a professional florist (find names and addresses in chapter 5, pages 242–244). If you're going to do the flowers yourself, try to make your arrangements as dramatic as possible. It's not the time for sweet little posies but for tall dramatic stems and branches in oversized containers. But for a smallish party at home you can buy lots of flowers inexpensively at markets. As I mentioned in chapter 5, the Flower Market in San Francisco is an amazing place, not only for the flowers themselves but for every kind of container you might need for them. In London I go to Nine Elms where containers are so cheap that I always end up buying far more than I need. There are buckets of every sort, huge vases in glass and ceramic—it sets the imagination going.

☞ *If you're going to have flowers on a dinner table, remember to keep them either quite low or very high (I've seen huge tall, thin vases with amazingly dramatic flowers emerging from the top) so that people can see each other across the table.*

Instead of flowers you could have big bowls of eggplants and oranges. I've seen ornamental cabbages, especially those small purple ones, displayed decoratively and looking wonderful. Nigella Lawson, I once read, likes big bowls of lemons.

At Christmas there's nothing like lots of black roses in dark vases—not cheap, I know, but very sophisticated. Otherwise get masses of one thing. Bunches of asparagus fern look good and in winter huge branches (and I mean huge: it's the flimsy approach that spoils it all) of leaves can be immensely effective. Bowls of pine cones don't cost much and look and smell wonderful.

I personally like to keep the table fairly plain with antique white linen cloths and big plain linen napkins but I do think at Christmas or for children's parties or themed parties, you can go a bit wild. At Christmas I always bring out a huge tartan cloth that I sewed up from lengths of fabric. It's a terrific background to a collection of red glass and pretty red and pink Ralph Lauren china.

And I love scented candles (though not in the dining room): a house should smell wonderful, too. There's a whole section on candles in chapter 5, page 245, but for parties my favorite smells of all time are Rigaud's Cyprès and Lorenzo Villoresi's Spezie.

INVITATIONS

For a grand party, I like invitations plain and classy on nice card with a classic typeface and thick creamy envelopes with tissue lining in a color of your choice. It's hard to beat Smythson's (877-769-8476 and at www.smythson.com), but there's no getting away from the fact that they're very expensive (that's what comes of being the leader in your field). Crane is a less expensive and very good alternative. If you're really savvy you can design your own at any printing outlet—FedEx Kinko's, for instance (www.fedex.com).

But there's nothing to stop you having funky invitations, or thinking up a special theme, or getting an artist or graphic designer friend to do something particular to you—it's your party after all. If you're a techie you can probably create your own on the computer. One friend makes her own Christmas cards every year, printing them out on clear, crinkly paper, and somehow they manage to seem cooler than anything shop bought.

> ☛ *Ideally invitations should go out at least six weeks before the event but for really serious parties (a big "O" birthday) when you really want all your favorite people to be there, send them out three, six, or even twelve months ahead of time.*

Some people ask calligraphists to write special invitations (for, say, a bar mitzvah or a wedding), which can look beautiful. I've known some people to send a balloon through the post you just blow up to read the invitation printed on it. Others have sent cute little records with songs inviting people to parties or DVDs, or even written on flip-flops for a beach party.

And while we're on the subject of invitations, guests should answer promptly. Imagine the angst of not knowing how many people to cater for.

SOME USEFUL ADDRESSES

Ever since the standards of food rose so dramatically catering has become a serious career opportunity and almost every small town and city offers endless choice. Key is finding one which suits your tastes and is prepared to provide precisely the service you're after. The grander ones usually only like to do, well, grand events. Often it's catering for the humbler events like family or friendly get-togethers that it's harder to find help for. Here are just some of the caterers that people I know and respect have found to be good.

Serena Bass, 404 West Thirteenth Street, New York 10014; 212-727-2257; www.serenabass.com.

Affairs to Remember, 680 Ponce de Leon Avenue NE, Atlanta, Georgia 30308; 404-872-7859; www.affairs.com.

Along Came Mary, 5265 West Pico Boulevard, Los Angeles 90019; 323-931-9082; www.alongcamemary.com.

East Meets West, 212 Old Colony Avenue, Boston 02127; 617-269-2662; www.eastmeetswestcatering.com.

Windows Catering Company, 5724 General Washington Drive, Alexandria, Virginia 22312; 703-519-3500; www.catering.com.

Music

Not, I have to say, my area of expertise (my almost-total ignorance of pop is a great gap in my education and something I'm determined to put right). If you're going to have dancing, live bands are wonderful. There are small ones all over the country that are thrilled to perform for not very large sums—you don't have to have Justin, J. Lo or any of the other mega-buck acts that hedge-fund managers seem to feel are essential for their jollifications. Otherwise track down a good DJ or ask your guests to bring along their favorite CDs. However, don't have the music so loud that nobody can hear anyone else speak.

The wrong music can ruin a party so choose it very, very carefully. If you want people to dance, you need some catchy dance music followed by some of the great classic dance music of all time. Go to a Virgin Megastore, which have personal shopping advisors who will guide you to the right music for you.

My young friends tell me that there are now wonderful compilations for good parties. They especially recommend the compilation from the Buddha Club in Paris and the Hotel Costes. Otherwise *After the Playboy Mansion* by Dmitri is, they tell me, loungy and cool. *Ultrachilled 01* is sophisticated and likely to appeal to those over fifty. All can be bought from www.amazon.com. These days there are people whom you can turn to for advice on how to fill the iPod (see page 325): just give them the scenario (over-fifties who want to dance; under-thirties who want something edgy, blues, jazz, whatever).

If you're after something more cultural, the music schools have trios and quartets, as well as singers, who are only too pleased to be asked to perform for not very large sums of money.

In case you're as ignorant about pop music as I am and want advice on what the great all-time pop records are so that you don't waste your time with junk, this is the list drawn up for me by James Brown, creator of *Loaded* magazine, former editor of *GQ* magazine, and currently editing *Quintessentially* magazine.

Rolling Stones: *Let It Bleed* and *Beggar's Banquet*
Lou Reed: *Transformer*
The Smiths: *The Queen Is Dead*
Marvin Gaye: *What's Going On*
Curtis Mayfield: *Superfly*
Bob Dylan: *Blonde on Blonde*
Michael Jackson: *Off the Wall*
Kate Bush: *Hounds of Love*
Patti Smith: *Horses*
Serge Gainsbourg: *Bonnie and Clyde*
Led Zeppelin: anything

DRINKS

If you're having a grand party with lots of people, you'll have to have somebody to help serve the drinks and then you can run more of an elaborate bar with fashionable mojitos and all the rest. If you're having a party at home and help is minimal, keep

---

Two Easy but Sophisticated Party Drinks

Simply pour a good, cold vodka over crushed ice and add lots of gorgeous pink pomegranate seeds—looks fabulous, tastes good.

Mix equal quantities of gin and Campari, plus half as much sweet red vermouth, with plenty of ice in a shaker. Add a thin slice of curled fresh orange peel.

---

the drinks simple. In chapter 6, I mention trying to offer some really delicious non-alcoholic drinks. Water is great but not very festive (though you do need to have lots of it on hand for those who simply get thirsty and don't only want alcohol). Try to offer something better than that. I was at a book launch once on a summer evening where the two drinks on offer were a refreshing melon drink (see the recipe on page 295) and champagne. Most people chose the melon drink.

Otherwise, I usually stick to champagne but have things like whiskey, vodka, and gin, as well as a good chilled white wine available for those who don't like champagne. Caterers tell me that you need to calculate for something like three-quarters of a bottle per person. Prosecco or some sparkling white wines are cheaper than champagne and some people actually prefer them. Some like mimosas (it's key not to add the orange juice—which must be really fresh—until just before serving) while others like Kir Royale (champagne with a little cassis), though speaking personally, if it's good champagne (and I'm not talking Dom Perignon, Bollinger, or Krug here: much too expensive for parties unless we're the Wall Street set, but I am talking something a cut above the horrible cheap sweet champagnes), I prefer it plain. Cooling champagne in bulk can be a problem. Check out www.elegantice.co.uk, which will deliver it in bulk and then you can cool lots of bottles in the bath.

If you're young and giving a party, you may find that at least half the guests prefer beer. Again use the bath to chill in quantity. If you're buying drink in bulk, most wine merchants will lend you enough glasses and they're usually of perfectly simple and acceptable design. They'll also supply ice in bulk.

As the evening wears on, offer lots of chances for non-alcoholic drinks: sparkling and still waters sprigged up with a little lemon and mint, really refreshing homemade lemonade or ginger beer can be fabulous.

Dinner Parties

My favorite sort of party. I personally never have enough time to spend hours making my table look amazing though I think it would be a lot of fun to do if one did (have enough time, that is). As you know, my tastes run to the classic look: white antique linen cloths, heavy plain white linen napkins, a selection of non-matching china and glass, set off by two huge hurricane lamps holding great cream candles. Those of you who are better organized can be more creative, coming up with endless different tables. Sherrie Bodie and Jan Grinling, two charming—and, it has to be said, dexterous—women *d'un certain âge* and clearly *d'un certain affluence*, are experts in the subject. They're nothing if not inventive—they have their minds firmly on the pennies and they don't go in for too much fancy work.

Here are a few of their tips. Always have a big generous cloth. If you don't have linen or antique ones, or you want to change the color scheme, they suggest you go to an Indian market for gorgeous saris, or yards of plain burlap, or curtain lining material (which they use under gauzy fabrics to give body and depth of color).

They use things like decorative hair bands as napkin rings and they pin little things like flowers, or old brooches and bits of glitter, to the band to make them look glamorous. They buy glass vases and bowls in assorted shapes from Ikea for anything between $2 and $7 each, or from department stores.

They create a lot of glamour with an all-black table. They start with a large black cloth, which they cover in mirrored table mats. Then come crystal plates (expensively from William Yeoward but Ikea has some at about $3 each). They fill little shot glasses with silver almonds to reflect the light and suggest dotting the table with glass tea lights with candles in them. Then around the table they scatter silver boxes, a collection of old decanter tops and other crystal bits and pieces—the idea being to catch and reflect as much light as possible. Napkins can be tied with black ribbon to finish the look.

They're very fond of centerpieces but they don't believe you always have to have flowers, lovely though they are. Try bowls of Christmas balls—either glass or silver, or a mixture of glass and silver, or fruits or vegetables. And don't forget candles— the most magical light of all (but they shouldn't be scented at a dinner table; keep them plain and creamy).

Food

I've already covered this in chapter 6. Food matters hugely but, as I said then, while it doesn't have to be elaborate, you can't get away with taking no trouble at all. What's right depends so much upon the season, the occasion and the guests.

I'm not keen on itsy-bitsy canapés though that is clearly what you need to serve if you're just having a drinks party. Suffice it to say that trends in this area change quite fast. At one point there was a rash of little Italian bites (tiny squares of ravioli, exquisite morsels of prosciutto and parmesan); then there was the trend for miniature portions of proletarian food made posh—fish and chips, eggs and bacon, hamburgers and the like; while as I write, Eastern still seems the reigning mood with tempting mouthfuls of sushi or teriyaki being served on equally exquisite pieces of Zen-like porcelain. I think only professional caterers can manage these things. If you're doing drinks at home and are catering yourself, it's best to keep it simple. I don't know anybody (except vegetarians) who doesn't like really, really good sausages or spiced nuts (see page 355 for recipe) or wonderful cheese straws. Even plain chunks of real parmesan are delicious, particularly if offered with a fragrant olive oil or balsamic vinegar to dip them into. Sometimes it's better to serve just a few rather more robust things—bruschetta with gravlax and mustard sauce, say, and some chicken satay on cocktail sticks.

Dinner-party food—particularly for those short of time—is covered pretty fully in chapter 6.

Buffet food, I find, is great fun to do. Lots of it can be prepared a little in advance. Once again generosity is the key—a huge platter of something simple like mozzarella, tomato and avocado, scattered with masses of basil and a really good olive oil and balsamic vinegar, looks wonderfully colorful and inviting. Many of the first courses in chapter 6 can be made in far larger quantities for buffets. Delia Smith's grilled vegetables with couscous (from *Delia Smith's Summer Collection*) make a terrific dish for a buffet lunch or supper and look brilliant too.

Some classic hot dishes make superb centerpieces. In the colder months there's nothing to beat a fantastic chili con carne served with baked potatoes, or an aromatic *boeuf en daube* (again with baked potatoes), or even a wonderful chicken or lamb tagine (with couscous or baked potatoes).

Sometimes it's fun to do a themed meal. For my father's eightieth birthday I did a buffet supper for about fifty people that homed in on his South African origins. I made a cold curried fish dish (easy to do and much, much more delicious than it sounds—it disappeared in a flash), and followed up with two classic South African dishes: *bobotie* (a South African version of moussaka in which the meat is slightly curried and mixed, when cooked, with a little bread soaked in milk, which may sound horrid but adds some creaminess to the texture, and then topped with a custard before being baked in the oven), served with a variety of chutneys, plus a meat and fruit curry. Any South African cookbook will have these recipes for they are probably the best-known indigenous dishes, reflecting the influence of Malay cooking. To finish, we had sorbets (brought in) made from tropical fruits—mango, passion fruit, pawpaw, guava, and the like. I can only say it went down a treat with some very sophisticated metropolitan types.

The idea can be adapted to almost any cuisine—Creole, French, Italian, Spanish, or anything else.

In summer there are some classic French dishes that make a really good centerpiece to a buffet lunch or supper—in particular a grand aioli, which consists of a huge, cold, cooked fish (classically cod but, in these more eco-conscious times, a freshly baked haddock would be equally lovely), surrounded by some tender, young, cooked vegetables (baby carrots, beans, asparagus, fennel, new potatoes, cauliflower, artichokes) and a vast pot of garlicky aioli in the middle. Or the Italian dish, *vitello tonnato*—cold, roasted veal sliced and served with a cold tuna-fish sauce. I also like a properly made coronation chicken (though not, please, with any pineapple anywhere near it), which is really just cooked chicken (best made with a boiling fowl from your butcher that has been gently poached), served in a lightly curried creamy sauce. And what's not to like about perfectly cooked chunky slices of pink filet of beef with a creamy horseradish or tartar sauce?

Add fresh salads, some good cheeses and patisserie, and you're there, though those who love cooking puddings can, of course, go to town.

You don't have to conjure up something different every time. We have friends, for instance, who always give us roast lamb on Sundays, others who always serve osso bucco (as it happens, one of my favorites, particularly when served with a classic risotto Milanese). There's quite a lot to be said for perfecting one dish and being known for it. I have a friend who makes the best cheesecake I know and I'd feel cheated if I turned up at her house and it wasn't offered.

For serving I find that antique china platters, picked up in antique shops and at antique fairs over the years, make the perfect background for cold dishes and salads.

Spiced Nuts

7 ounces mixed shelled nuts of your choice
   (almonds, hazelnuts, cashews, pistachios, pecans, etc.)

1 tablespoon chopped fresh rosemary
   (discarding the stalks)

¼ teaspoon cayenne pepper

1½ tablespoons brown sugar

1 teaspoon salt

½ teaspoon walnut or olive oil

Preheat the oven to 325° F. Mix all the ingredients together and spread out on a baking sheet. Bake for 10 minutes. Remove from the oven, stir, turning them over, and return to the oven to bake for another 10 minutes. Cool on the tray. When cold, store in an airtight container for up to a week. (*With thanks to Renate Gunn.*)

CHRISTMAS

Christmas, unless you're so organized that you've bought your presents in the January sales or in September and have them all wrapped by October, is stressful for most of us, but especially for those with jobs and precious little help. Some things can't (or rather, shouldn't) be delegated—such as getting your secretary to buy your husband's Christmas present—but many can. Help is out there and it comes in varying packages—some very expensive, some surprisingly reasonable. Here's a guide to just some of what is available.

Presents

I don't think buying gifts should be handed over lock, stock, and barrel to somebody else (who else would know that your husband hates a certain shade of blue, or that the son and heir already has everything Bob Dylan ever wrote), but advice and suggestions are always useful (the stores usually know what the hot children's toys are), while wrapping, packing and delivery can all be safely delegated. If you need more ideas on presents there are lots to be found in chapter 7.

Stores are realizing more and more that personal service is the key to buying the customers' loyalty and so personal shoppers are on the increase. Bloomingdales, for instance, has a team of gift gurus. You can simply turn up at the information desk and ask for one, pose your questions (what's the best laptop case, what's the hot handbag) and you'll be directed to the right department. For more personal advice, book into their personal-shopping service. Free gift-wrapping is available all through the store but, though very attractive, it will announce its Bloomingdale's origins.

Stockings are supposed to be fun and they usually are but oh, the stress. I remember well sitting up until one or two in the morning, wrapping every single satsuma and paperback personally. Nowadays small stores will often take over the job but the downside is you have less control over the contents.

If your time in the boardroom doesn't leave enough time for wrapping or store visiting, there's an array of the new breed of lifestyle or concierge services that will do it for you. The downside is that you have to pay a membership fee and while they can nearly always solve most problems, the price isn't cheap. The upside is that you can describe exactly what it is you're after and leave it to them to track it down. These services are particularly useful if you're desperate because the ten-year-old has to have this year's hot present and all the shops have sold out, or there'll be tears beside the tree if you haven't found the right Chloé blouse.

Quintessentially (www.quintessentially.com), for instance, has an annual membership fee but that gives you access to a whole host of services. It now has a special department called Quintessentially Gifts, with a small army of personal shoppers who will do the shopping for you—for a fee. It can also organize tree delivery and collection, as well as send somebody to dress the tree.

Consider It Done (888-860-3663; www.consideritdone .com) charges $2,500 a month for twenty hours' worth of services, if you commit to a contract. If you need more hours you can buy them on an ad hoc basis. If you're pushed only at Christmas, you can hire them for $1,200 for eight hours of labor—they'll order the turkey, decorate the house or the tree, send off the Christmas cards or search for presents. You choose.

Trees and Decorations

If you've young children and choosing your very own tree together from the market—or the forest—is part of the fun, good. If not, get it delivered. Choose a Fraser fir if you don't want to clog up the vacuum cleaner.

The Christmas Tree Association (636-449-5070 and at www.christmastree.org). Their Web site lists suppliers of Christmas trees all over the country.

A Fresh Christmas Tree (616-975-7590 and at www.afreshchristmastree.com) will deliver trees, wreaths and garlands nationwide and for an extra charge will provide simple decorations in the shape of little bows and ornaments.

Macy's usually has a ready-designed tree, which means a package of tastefully chosen decorations, and it will deliver the (artificial) tree plus all the non-breakable baubles and decorations, which you then have to attach yourself.

www.greenpointtrees.com will deliver your tree, install it and light it, but only, sadly, for those who live in the New York metropolitan area. The site www.spmistletoe.com will deliver boxes of mistletoe. All over the country, there are professionals who will come and hang lights, garland the tree or the house and after the celebrations are over they'll take them all down and store them until next year rolls round—expensive but for the busy, busy set, well worth it; you can find a local professional at www.christmasdecor.net.

Christmas Food

The trick here is not to aim at perfection. Culinary pyrotechnics are not essential at Christmas and if you're a budding Wolfgang Puck you can leave the fancy cooking for another time. Order ahead the very best organic turkey (or sirloin, goose, whatever your family fancies), ham, and smoked salmon from companies such as West Wind Farms (www.grass organic.com) or Diamond Organics (www.diamondorganics .com), and then do the rest of it the easy way. Fine cheeses can be ordered from www.cowgirlcreamery.com. You can order everything online, if you can master the technology—remember that Peapod (www.peapod.com) and Safeway (www.safeway .com) are the busy woman's patron saints—or go to the best food store near you. Buy already-prepared brussels sprouts, potatoes ready to roast (unless you have your own patent recipe), preprepared roasted parsnips, white sauce, pudding, and all the rest from the good stores. Save your time and keep your nerves in good shape so that you can enjoy your family and friends. Add cream to the white sauce, a tad more brandy to the brandy butter (the traditional accompaniment to the pudding), masses of herbs to the vegetables, sprinkle some nutmeg on the brussels sprouts, and toss them with caramelized canned chestnuts, and you're there.

☞ AND DON'T FORGET . . . the loo. Always have lovely soaps and good hand lotions available, as well as small piles of nice old-fashioned plain linen or huckaback hand towels.

GOOD MANNERS

Manners are an age-old condition of the civilized mind, in order to have a system of behavior which prevents human contact from sliding into chaos and old night. The primitive peoples of Africa that I have known have wonderful manners and the most courteous and orderly forms of debate. One of the most significant things for me in Dante's

> *great journey down into Hell and up into Heaven*
> *was that in Hell there was an absence of good*
> *manners; when he emerged and arrived in Purga-*
> *tory he was amazed how grace and courtesy be-*
> *tween the spirits he encountered were already*
> *present, and increased with a breathtaking and*
> *inspiring acceleration as he neared paradise.*
>
> —A WALK WITH A WHITE BUSHMAN,
> LAURENS VAN DER POST

Good manners, in my book, real manners, the sort that are about an inner grace, have nothing to do with where you put the soup spoons or whether you say "toilet" or "loo." Real manners are about considering other people. Certain formalities exist to smooth the path and give us guidelines, but at the end of the day the matter is very simple: well-mannered people are never rude to others, or hurtful, and never do anything that makes other people feel awkward or small.

I well remember being at a party when a male guest had inadvertently got the dress code wrong and turned up in a turtleneck sweater when everybody else was in suits. He was welcomed in by his host and introduced all round. Some ten minutes later the host appeared—wearing a turtleneck sweater. Now that's what I call real manners, where the host wanted immediately to make a guest feel at home.

Then I remember being at a lunch given by the mayor of Avignon. The first course consisted of lovely fat spears of white asparagus served with hollandaise sauce. I picked mine up in my fingers, but it wasn't until I'd eaten the first one that I looked around and saw that everybody else was eating them with a knife and fork. Scarlet with embarrassment, I turned to my host and explained that in England everybody eats asparagus with their fingers. My host had an immediate response.

"*Tout le monde les mange avec la bouche* [Everyone eats them with their mouth]," was his sweet reply. That is what I call real manners.

So while saying "please" and "thank you" matter up to a point, true manners, really graceful behavior, means never being unkind, and never doing or saying anything to make anybody else feel small. It involves putting others at ease at all times and considering their feelings.

I must say that I'm not much enamored of what sometimes passes for manners in so-called sophisticated and socially elevated circles. I observe—regularly—at apparently smart parties the kind of rudenesses that an African in a rural village would be ashamed of. It isn't, in my view, decent behavior to blank people to whom you have been introduced several times but whom you deem to be somehow uninteresting or beneath you. No African in his traditional society would ever do this. Acknowledging the existence of another human is a critical form of showing respect—and kindness. Yet this happens every day at grand gatherings.

At dinner parties, if you're lucky enough to be invited to them and you accept, then it seems to me that you should sing for your supper, which includes taking an interest in your neighbor. I have sat through many a dinner party where I have taken a deep interest in the intricacies of my (male) neighbor's work/life/hobbies but have not had a single enquiry as to the nature of my own concerns—the implicit attitude being that they couldn't possibly be of such absorbing interest as his. I've never quite known how to deal with this but a friend, to whom it happened recently, listened dutifully for a long time, punctuated the monologue with suitable questions and finally, exasperated, turned to her neighbor and said: "Since there is clearly not a single thing of interest that I can tell you about myself, I will bid you goodnight"—and with that she turned on her heel. I'm sure the neighbor to this day will not have the smallest clue as to why she behaved as she did.

I myself am rather guilty on the punctuality front but I mind it, think it's rude, and berate myself continually for not always being on time. Being late implies that the other person's time is of less value than your own. For meetings and in one's social life, I think it's important to turn up when you've said you would, most particularly when it's a formal dinner and precise numbers matter. Unless you really are ill, it's seriously bad manners to cancel the day of. Dinners in cities tend to start on the late side but arrive no more than twenty minutes after the time you were asked for and don't overstay your welcome.

I think how you dress matters when it comes to dinner and party invitations. Okay, if you're very young and you're all gathering for supper in somebody's apartment, dress codes are entirely superfluous. Or rather, you'll know what they are and you'll probably have the right pair of jeans in your wardrobe as well as the au courant pair of shoes. You'll know exactly how *déshabillé* it is currently fashionable to be and how much glamming up is part of the scene. And anyway it's just as much a cause of embarrassment to overdress—to turn up as if you're expecting a banquet when your friends had scrambled egg in mind—as to underdress.

Invitations these days usually specify some kind of sartorial code. It may vary from casual (rather a bummer, that one) to black tie, white tie, informal, or "festive" (even more of a bummer). If you're stumped, it's best to be quite straightforward and simply call and ask. What is unforgivable, in my view, is for the hostess to so arrange things that all her guests turn up looking ridiculous (having been asked to dress "gypsy" or "decadent" or "over the top") while she swans around, elegantly and minimally chic. I remember being invited on a very small and privileged press trip and told to bring just jeans and casual wear, only to find my tall, slim and beautiful companion had packed a different glam outfit for every single evening. That is very poor manners in my view.

I think there's nothing better than a hand-written thank-you letter to follow up a dinner, lunch or opera invitation and the sooner you write it, the better. The longer you leave it, the more time it takes because you have to make it more fulsome, more eloquent and probably include a bunch of flowers to boot. I'm not a big fan of thank-yous by e-mail—a growing modern habit—unless it be for something like a casual girly lunch. I like taking small presents to dinner parties and bigger ones when you are asked to stay overnight, for weekends or holidays (see chapter 7).

How to Deal with Some Modern Dilemmas

Q. You're on a low-GI (no starch, no sugar) or a wheat-free diet, and you're invited over to a friend's house for dinner. Do you expect them to tailor their meal to your needs or just hope for the best?

A. If it's a diet for serious health reasons (allergies, cholesterol, diabetes), call well in advance and explain. Women today understand these things. Otherwise eat your way around the plate as best you can. Do not call with peculiar requests an hour before dinner begins.

Q. You've just put away the pudding plates and are serving up the coffee when a couple of your guests start offering a line of cocaine. Can you ask them to stop?

A. Certainly. They're the ones breaching the rules.

Q. Most people hate smoking these days. A guest in your house lights up. Can you ask them not to smoke?

A. My own view is that tobacco isn't illegal (like cocaine), and if you've asked a smoker to your house, then you should grin and bear it. A host's duty is to make his guests' stay enjoyable and comfortable. Manners, though, are reciprocal and these days, the considerate guest who finds himself in the home of a nonsmoker usually takes himself and his cigarettes outside before he lights up.

Q. We're getting married and we've got most of the things we need for the house. Is it okay to ask wedding guests for money?

A. No, it's not. If you've got all you need, ask guests to make a contribution to charity. Otherwise ask for something that nobody ever has too much of—wine or books, to name but two.

Q. We often go out to dinner with other couples but, as I never drink, I feel we're always paying more than our share of the bill. Is there any way round this?

A. Only by dining alone. There's something indescribably small and mean about people splitting hairs over the cost of shared meals.

Q. Should a woman always pay her share of bills on a date?

A. If it's a first date, and he's asked you out as well as chosen the restaurant/theater/opera, I would let him pay. After that you can offer to pay your share. Once you're going steady you're presumably up for sharing bills. If you're richer than him, you should sometimes treat him completely.

Q. Is it okay to send invitations out by e-mail?

A. If it's an impromptu informal barbecue on a Sunday or a sudden invitation to a theater, yes. If it's a proper party, no—send a stiffy some six weeks at least before the big event.

Q. I always get stuck at parties with the most boring man on the planet. How do I get rid of him politely?

A. You take him over to meet somebody else and introduce him, saying, 'I want to introduce you two to each other,' and then you move quickly away. If your or his glass is empty, you use that as an excuse to ask for a refill and quietly move over to another group while he fetches it. When he returns you're deep in conversation with somebody else.

Q. Is it okay to break off a relationship by e-mail or text message?

A. You're seriously asking? No, no, no. It's cowardly, small, and weasely. Do it face-to-face.

Q. If a guest arriving for dinner brings a bottle, is it impolite not to serve it?

A. No. Guests understand that you've probably planned the wine beforehand and, anyway, one bottle isn't going to go far if you're having more than four people round.

Q. Is it ever all right to complain?

A. Of course. The key is to keep your voice beautifully soft and polite while you utter the killer complaint. Do not raise your voice, do not shout, just say in the most gracious tones, "Please never treat me like that ever again." Or whatever else it is you wish to complain about.

And Finally . . .

A Few Things
I Wish I'd Known Long Ago

I wish I'd known how wonderful it was to be twenty, thirty, forty. . . .

You can't please all of the people all of the time.

Don't be too afraid of making an enemy—sometimes courage and honesty require it.

Never take offense—only small people take offense.

If it doesn't fit in the shop, it's not going to fit when you get it home.

The things you worry about are almost never the things that happen.

Never have anything to do with men who carry little purses.

It's better to clean and tidy less and read more.

Never go out with a man who doesn't make you laugh.

You can't change most people. Don't expect them to give what they are unable to give.

Don't do anything grudgingly. If you're going to do it, however much you hate it, you might as well do it well.

Never be stingy with tips. It always leaves one feeling lousy.

You can't have too many sexy shoes.

Sexiness has nothing to do with being size 2 or looking like Sienna Miller.

Use the things you love every day. It's never worth saving things for a special occasion.

It's always worth reading—and learning—poetry.

A great haircut is worth any number of new dresses.

Never buy anything because "It's bound to come in useful."

Never buy anything that you don't love or that isn't absolutely right.

Acknowledgments

I would like to thank all those many editors on *The Sunday Times, Financial Times,* and *The Times* who have encouraged me through the years, given me a platform, sent me off to weird and wonderful places, and generally allowed me to have more fun than sometimes seemed decent. Also, huge thanks to Eleanor Birne and Nikki Barrow at John Murray, whose idea this book was in the first place. In addition I would like to thank my American editor, Courtney Napoles, of Da Capo for her inestimable insights into the American way of life and Georgia Feldman for her elegant art direction.

Index

LUCIA VAN DER POST, the founding editor of the *Financial Times' How to Spend It* magazine, writes regularly about style and design for the *Financial Times, The Times* of London, and many other newspapers and magazines. A mother and grandmother, she lives in London.